RED LIGHT GREEN LIGHT

Preventing Teen Pregnancy

RED LIGHT, GREEN LIGHT: Preventing Teen Pregnancy

Portrayals in this book are composite sketches with no personal reference to a prevention, pregnancy, or parenting story. This is done to protect confidentiality.

Published by Summer Kitchen Press, Helena, Montana.

Library of Congress Catalog Card Number: 96-70009
Library of Congress Cataloging In Publication Data: Pending

ISBN: 0-9653647-0-4

Cover and Illustrations by Joel Nakamura
Cover Design by Annette Finstad
Book Design, Typesetting by Summer Kitchen Press

Distributed by: Summer Kitchen Press, 314 Chaucer Street, Helena, Montana 59601.

ATTENTION COLLEGES AND UNIVERSITIES, ADOLESCENT HEALTH CARE PROFESSIONALS, SOCIAL SERVICE ORGANIZATIONS, CHURCHES, FOUNDATIONS AND CORPORATIONS: Quantity and wholesale discounts are available. For more information please contact the author at 1-800-418-5237 or write: Summer Kitchen Press, 314 Chaucer Street, Helena, Montana 59601.

First Edition

Manufactured in the United States of America

DEDICATION

This book is dedicated to my husband, Steve,
Our sons, Jason and Joshua, and
Laura Christensen Colberg and Heather Humphrey,
To my parents, Melvin and Irja Ollila,
To my sister and her husband, Kathy-Dennis Ohlund,
To my brother and his son, Rod and Christopher Ollila,
And to my sister-in-law Marjorie Colberg Meyer, my most candid editor.

TABLE OF CONTENTS

CREDITS

Illustrations copyrighted and used by permission of Joel Nakamura, Illustrator

Page 5,   "The Mating Game"- An illustration about primordial reproductive instincts.

Page 11, "Prophecy"

Page 29, "Skull Man With Mask"

Page 37, "Have A Heart, Give A Hand" - Expressing the mandala.

Page 39, "Nativity"

Page 62, "AIDS and the Theatre" - AIDS decimating the theatrical community while giving rise to creative playwriting.

Page 72, "Looking For Mr. Right"- Computer dating.

Page 81, "Unnamed"

Page 91, "Time banking"

Page 47, Rathus Assertiveness Schedule copyrighted material used by permission of its author, Spencer A. Rathus.

ACKNOWLEDGMENTS

A variety of experiences molded this perspective on teen pregnancy prevention. The most global contributions are from the lives of women in Afghanistan where my husband, Steve, and I spent two years in the Peace Corps. This experience gave us the opportunity to enter the lives of the Afghan women who were veiled by the *chaderi* and protected by the compound wall. Teen males filled the nursing classes I taught in Lashkar Gah, Afghanistan. Their wives and families needed a midwife and often I became that helper because I was a nurse with maternity room experience. These Afghan women were the property of the men. First they belonged to the father. At marriage, the bride became the groom's property upon payment of the bride price. The wives were young. Some were still in puberty and experiencing their first pregnancy at twelve to fourteen years of age. The prevalence of disease and scarcity of proper medical attention allowed only an estimated sixty percent of pregnancies to reach full term gestation and survive beyond the first five years of life.

Peace Corps training took place at a migrant labor camp in Weld County, Colorado. The perplexities of another culture contributed to the need for preventing teen pregnancy. The migrant families were large and about half the pregnant women in my prenatal classes were teenagers. These teens were married and worked in the sugar beet fields until delivery. The Catholic faith was a strong spiritual bond holding the migrant families together through what seemed insurmountable odds.

A third contribution to this view on prevention is from the Northern European culture of my heritage. My mother is from Finland and my father is also Finnish. Both family homesteads are in New York Mills, Minnesota, acknowledged in old history books as "the largest Finnish stronghold in the United States." My mother was never ashamed or bashful about discussing how things were in "the old country." Young Finnish men and women often married after they were pregnant; this was not shameful or unexpected. It was practical and acceptable. The long arctic winters of Northern Finland limited travel of the itinerant cleric who did funerals, weddings, and christenings in the little villages of his pastorate. The dead kept cold until proper burial, the young kept warm as almost married folks, and the babies born after the last clerical visit were blessed with a name when spring thaws permitted travel of the minister.

A fourth important contribution to the views expressed in *Red Light, Green Light* is through work as a high school nurse. Parents and the pregnant and parenting students of the support groups helped create this book. They will recognize representations of their lives and pregnancies. However, to preserve anonymity and confidentiality, all narratives are composites with no reference to a specific prevention, pregnancy, or parenting story.

The last and most important contributions to this book are marriage to my husband, Steve, and the birth, raising, and joy-filled sharing of life with our sons, Jason and Joshua. Steve, with his experience in computer graphics and desk-top publishing, has been a constant teacher and helper. With a grateful heart I thank these people. It is my intent that the viewpoint of the reader is enriched by other perspectives to consider as we explore preventing teen pregnancy. **All ideas expressed in this book are the responsibility of the author.**

OVERVIEW

Red Light, Green Light helps teens by educating their peers, counselors, parents, grandparents, health care providers, teachers, ministers, and group leaders about teen sexuality. This book discusses important issues of teen pregnancy prevention. *Red Light, Green Light* is organized into modules instead of chapters because each section describes specific interchangeable activities. Ideally these modules are used when small groups of teens are taught to help each other. However, the interactive nature of *Red Light, Green Light* allows one caring adult to mentor a youngster with this book as a program guide.

Red Light, Green Light emphasizes preventing teen pregnancy by understanding adolescent social behaviors. Preteens and teens will benefit from this book as much as the adolescent whose social maturity is hastened by pregnancy. For example, this book shows the need for healthy messages about sexuality long before adolescence. When puberty arrives, the teen has a sense of what makes him or her tick. Adolescents develop the confidence to accept the changes the teen years bring, to use or to reject the models of adult behaviors that they see, to express feelings, to affirm differences among people, and to accept their own imperfections and life's unfairness.

Teens in our society are all in similar situations. Nonpregnant and pregnant young people alike find that they are both working on dating and relationships. They are deciding boundaries and whether or not to be sexually active. They are both concerned about academic, vocational, and extracurricular activities so they will have a future with good job opportunities. They are separating from their families and becoming independent and self-sufficient. All teens are making choices about growing up without the crippling effects of alcohol, tobacco, and other drugs. However, there is no uniformity in the preparation of teens to face these changes. Some teens have strong support from families, friends, and community while others have no one to provide emotional stability.

"Here Is How I Can Use This Book."

Red Light, Green Light studies the concerns of teen pregnancy to gather information about preventing a pregnancy in the first place. Parents are encouraged to use the book because they are the first and most important "line of defense" in teen pregnancy prevention. The concepts used in *Red Light, Green Light* were developed by working with pregnant teens who had a low rate of repeat pregnancies in their teen years. The three main goals of that program were to: 1) promote maternal, paternal, and child health and well-being, 2) complete high school, and 3) prevent a second pregnancy. These three goals are common to teens who are not pregnant and become important to the prevention of first pregnancies as well. See the "Resource Guide" on page 115.

Red Light, Green Light consists of modules or units based on counseling techniques and shaped by experience with groups of teens. A vignette or composite sketch introduces each unit. The modules are interchangeable; however, the present order considers group work as described by Marianne and Gerald Corey in their book, *Groups: Process and Practice*. Modules One through

Four introduce the topics of sexuality, individual counseling, and group formation. This initial stage is called *forming*.

Modules Five and Six introduce the central theme of the mandala and the importance of building self-worth and making personal spiritual choices. The group builds trust and finds an identity of its own; these modules represent the group process of the transitional stage called *norming*.

Modules Seven through Seventeen are brief presentations of serious concerns that impact teen sexuality and the commitment to investigate behaviors that prevent teen pregnancy. Members may not agree with each other. These modules together represent the working stage of group process called *storming*.

By the time group closure or the final stage of Module Eighteen occurs, *conforming* is evident. Group members respect each other's ideas and differences and know when to support "agreeing to disagree."

The aim of *Red Light, Green Light* is to present a program that serves the whole personality of the teenager. For instance, the modules on puberty and the health questionnaire will serve many adolescents and answer their questions about sexuality. The module on gestation will be more suitable to the teen and her partner who face a teen pregnancy and are curious about its meaning. Modules on pregnancy and child-rearing also give nonpregnant teens and their parents a chance to vicariously view teen pregnancy with the intent of preventing it. For all readers, this book presents information about adolescent sexuality with the purpose of skill-building and problem-solving.

> **... this program does not depend on a lot of money to be effective. It is flexible in times of unpredictable funding.**

The vignette at the beginning of each module expresses the main teen concern discussed in the unit. Use the body of the module as a workbook with teens either individually or in a group. Move through each section, and note the attached handouts. Use these handouts for individual counseling or as a student workbook for group sessions. A goal statement that helps the reader focus on the significance of each module follows the vignette. The objectives are statements of purpose that show the measured steps to reach the goal. The method clarifies the purpose. Each module closes with practical questions that increase the reader's awareness so they can evaluate the effectiveness of the unit for their needs. Answers to some questions may require investigation of resources in one's community.

Finally, this program does not depend on a lot of money to be effective. It is flexible in times of unpredictable funding. One person can oversee a small program on a low budget. In times of low funding, a person depends on the help of volunteers from community agencies who can serve as guest speakers for select units. *Red Light, Green Light's* approach to reaching teens represents an adaptation of materials developed for use in the school, the church, the community, in private counseling practice, and as a one-on-one mentoring program.

MODULE ONE
INTRODUCTION

"The Dilemma"

Lana's quick footsteps, a toss, and a thud signal the arrival of the newspaper and the start of a new day. Clare turns over in the sweet, warm darkness of her bed covers, hugging the blanket around her shoulders just as Bob Edward's reassuring voice from the small clock radio takes the edge off any bad news coming over the six o'clock airwaves.

Clare slides out of bed and blindly pulls on her jogging suit not thinking about the morning routine just then. Downstairs the coffeepot chortles for ten minutes and is almost done. Taking three swigs of the warm, brown liquid, Clare heads into the darkness of another short December day. Lana's footsteps in the snow are a comfort to Clare; nothing can happen in a neighborhood where kids do their early morning paper route and puppies pad along faithfully beside their young masters. Lana never misses a day; she is as constant as the six o'clock news.

Then it stops. Lana has not been on her paper route for more than a week. The paper quits coming at its appointed hour; Saturday it nearly misses delivery at all. One could phone the *Denver Post* for retribution, but that isn't the point. We are worried about Lana; it isn't like her to quit a job and not give us, her fan club, adequate notice. Finally, on a Sunday night two weeks later, there is a soft knock on the front door. There is Lana, in her red Mackinaw, looking drawn and pale with dark circles around her eyes.

"Where have you been?" Clare asks half angrily, half caringly. "Were you sick? Have you quit?" Too many questions tumble out so fast Lana cannot answer them and crumbles into a small, sobbing heap as she answers. "I can't be a paper girl. I'm pregnant. What am I going to do? Where am I going to go?" Tears fill Clare's eyes too. It sounds ridiculous, a pregnant paper girl, it can't be. "What will you *do*?"

> **"I can't be a paper girl. I'm pregnant. What am I going to do?"**

The way Lana got through those tough years of raising a child, going to college, and coming to terms with her loneliness were avoidable. If she had delayed pregnancy, Lana would not carry the grieving of lost teen years and hastened adult responsibilities. She would not shelter her first-born child whose feelings of abandonment are never relieved by a support check.

Our society's dilemma of teen pregnancy is an expression of many factors. First, a combination of parental permissiveness, earlier teen maturation and mobility, and the availability of birth control have promoted sexual experimentation as early as the preteen years. This experimentation coupled with invincibility, a notion so prevalent in teens, is an explosive mixture that allows untimely pregnancies to occur. Peer group influence and the desire to appear intimate increase risk-taking behavior.

Second, the complexity of our society leads to high expectations of our youth. Many times teen pregnancy is viewed as a "shame" not deserving of remedy. The pregnant adolescent is easy to identify because pregnancy cannot be hidden; it is noticeable. The teen fathers who walk in support of their partners are easy to identify as well. If an adolescent chooses abortion she may not be easy to identify, but she feels the defeat without the acknowledgment and support that are important to healing.

Another factor, the cost of material goods and the attitude that consumerism engenders, does not allow much time for enjoying children. Instead of increasing quality time with children, materialism has become the driving force behind the phenomenon of the unsupervised "latch-key kid." Economic realities are a double challenge to the pregnant teen who has extra expenses without the skills needed for jobs that offer higher wages and a better standard of living. Welfare programs often meet the financial needs of the pregnant youngster whose family is already beset with poverty. The downside of this financial relief is that dependence permanently erodes a teen's self-confidence.

Fourth, the reality of dysfunctional families increases unintended pregnancies. Poor adult role modeling leaves young people confused about their boundaries and role expectations. The lack of caring adult supervision increases the chance of rape and incest. And the grooming of children to early sexualization by predatory adults increases the likelihood of teen pregnancy.

Teen pregnancy will personally change the lives of two million young people, their babies, and their families this year. Teen pregnancy will be as close as your immediate or extended family. Or it may be removed to the girl or boy in your neighborhood or as remote as a stark headline to conjecture about as you read the morning daily.

> **. . . people are committed to preventing teen pregnancy because they want to nurture youth in their birthright to a wholesome and carefree adolescence.**

The goal of this book is to investigate the nature of adolescent pregnancy to learn what prevents a pregnancy in the first place. The reader, be he or she a teenager, a parent, a grandparent, a teacher, a health care professional, a counselor, a minister, or a youth leader, becomes aware of real life concerns faced by teens. More importantly, these people are committed to preventing teen pregnancy because they want to nurture youth in their birthright to a wholesome and carefree adolescence.

"What's Your Point?"

Teenagers do not operate from mission statements and strategies as do today's corporations, churches, and school districts. Teens ask, "What's your point?"; their vernacular asks for the same accountability in an abbreviated way. To answer, the goal of *Red Light, Green Light* is to promote prevention of pregnancy by understanding teen sexuality and enabling teens to find meaningful answers for themselves.

GOAL: To empower teens by providing advocacy, health enrichment, spiritual resiliency, and group support.

Objective One: Assess the validity and reliability of statistics available for investigating the need to reach and to teach teens before pregnancy occurs.

Objective Two: Identify adolescents who need physical, emotional, social, and spiritual support.

Objective Three: Help adolescents develop their ideas, talents, and peer support for themselves and other teens.

Objective Four: Explore family values and an interactive educational model that promotes the prevention of first teen pregnancies.

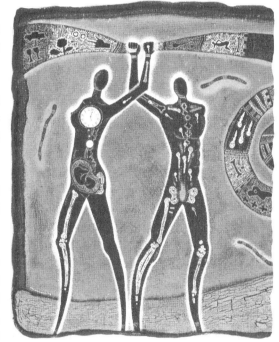

Objective Five: Establish pregnancy prevention and support program guidelines that foster academic and vocational success and promote graduation from high school.

Objective Six: Encourage community alliances that enrich the physical, mental, social, and spiritual health of teens.

METHOD: Have you noticed that annual reports of teen pregnancy rates in the United States have not changed for the last two decades? From publications by the Alan Guttmacher Institute, that deal with the concerns of teen pregnancy, to articles from nursing and counseling journals or your local newspaper, the introductory statement about teen pregnancy often reads, "More than one million teenagers in the United States become pregnant each year."

This fact infers that teen pregnancy is of monumental concern as a societal issue and the problem is not becoming smaller. We see that this seven-digit figure denotes only the pregnant female. We can quickly double that number if we consider that for every pregnant female there is a pregnant male, though he may not be a teenager.

The "Youth Risk Behavior Survey," a standardized questionnaire administered to randomly selected groups of high school adolescents, is used to collect data in thirty-three states. This survey is the only standardized instrument used across the United States that generates information about teen sexual behaviors and related-health outcomes. The survey has been repeated in the selected schools every two years since 1988.

Every state contributes their information on adolescent pregnancy to the Center for the Study of Social Policy and the Annie E. Casey Foundation who publish *The Kids Count Data Book*. This data book includes statistics on teen pregnancy and the following nine high risk corollaries: 1) percentage of low birth weight babies, 2) infant mortality rate, 3) child death rate, 4) juvenile violent crime arrest rate, 5) percentage of dropouts from high school, 6) percentage of teens not in school and not in labor force, 7) teen violent death rate, 8) percent children in poverty, and 9) percentage of children in single parent homes. See "Current Statistics" on page 114.

Red Light, Green Light acknowledges these risk factors and offers a teen pregnancy prevention program that empowers adolescents by providing advocacy, health enrichment, spiritual resiliency, and group support. Goals of the youth, their parents, and their leaders are in tandem; they are to: 1) promote good physical, mental, and spiritual health in teens, 2) encourage graduation and vocational success, and 3) foster prevention of pregnancy in the teen years.

The **first successful strategy** of the program is that teens and adults together have examined the treatment of teen pregnancy to learn about prevention.   From this study has grown a **teen pregnancy prevention program** that addresses decreasing, delaying, preventing, or deterring pregnancy in the adolescent years.

The **second successful strategy** of *Red Light, Green Light* is that it embraces reaching and supporting the spiritual needs of the identified students. Carl Jung in his work as a psychotherapist talked about the mandala or "magic circle" which represents the indwelling spiritual core in the life of each person.   Adapting Jung's ideas to our human desire for spiritual wholeness allows sharing of emotional and spiritual concerns.   Participants investigate their family values, patterns of emotional expression, and indwelling spiritual core. They do not assume or presume another person's emotional or spiritual connection.

An example of this spirituality lies in the Native American youth whose way of communication with their extended family or tribe is through the "talking circle." Each of us carries an example of spiritual wholeness. Any time we acquaint ourselves with another person we see another heritage that broadens our world view and permits us to see another individual's spiritual similarities and differences.

Red Light, Green Light never separates the concern about untimely pregnancy from the male's responsibility. Our hope is to include the male soon enough to plan for fatherhood and for nurturing relationships with his partner and their child. Module Fourteen, entitled "Male Responsibility and Father Bonding," emphasizes the importance of including men in the discussion of preventing teen pregnancy.

QUESTIONS FOR CONSIDERATION:

1)   Name different societal indicators that accompany increasing teen pregnancy rates. How do your state and local statistics of teen pregnancy compare with statistics across the nation?

2)   What agencies and publications provide continuing information about these indicators in your community? Are statistics gathered in a way that is valid and reliable? How are teens involved in contributing their ideas as statistics are collected?

3)   Community networking and alliances are important to the prevention of teen pregnancy. Identify, contact, and discuss the mission of each community service that addresses teen sexuality and pregnancy prevention. Make a directory for use with teens in your home, your church, and your school.

4)   Of the services listed in question three, which ones are available to males?

5)   Identify people in the community who would be part of a speaker's bureau to discuss teen pregnancy prevention.   How would one solicit parental support for this venture?

6)   Identify obstacles to working with pregnant and parenting teens. What obstacles come from the adolescents? How does one enlist the support of the administrator in the school setting? What obstacles might one expect from the community? Parents? School faculty and staff?

7)   Identify strategies appropriate to your community for dealing with these obstacles.

8)   Who are the most appropriate people to serve on a committee that investigates curricula or programs of teen pregnancy prevention? Use the "Resource Guide" on page 115.

9)   How does one involve teens in decision-making about teen pregnancy prevention without breaching confidentiality?

10)   What is the meaning of "agreeing to disagree?"

MODULE TWO
PUBERTY

"Red Birds And Green Bees"

Five minutes on the streets of Kabul, Afghanistan, piqued a curiosity about the hawkers on each street corner. The small stands sold exactly the same items: combs, Moslem amulets, plastic pens, *shajuk* or gum, and condoms. The *shajuk* and condoms were favorite items of the grade school boys.

We were Peace Corps volunteers committed to work in this distant and mysterious country halfway around the globe from our homeland. Veiled women wove in and out of the crowded bazaars shopping with just as much enthusiasm as any American woman. The vendors and shopkeepers were all men. Even on the hottest summer days the men wore pajama-like outfits covered by a full-length flowing robe. They covered their head with an embroidered skullcap surrounded by a turban. The turban had a variety of uses. Wet or dry, it was a towel to wipe a beaded brow. It became a basket to carry rice and fruit home from the market. The turban was a rug to kneel upon when offering daily prayers to Allah. It became a cradle for a sleeping infant, or a blanket for an older child as he slept under a tree while a vigilant father waited for his *bachem* to awake.

We rested under a tree as well, watching the banter of boys racing home after school by way of the bazaar. Shouting *"ballou, ballou"*, they went by, sharing the condoms they had just purchased from a nearby vendor. Boys will be boys! And this raucous group sabotaged our best efforts to advocate birth control. They used the condoms as water balloons!

In America this would be a "teachable moment," meaning that a parent would teach to a youngster's natural curiosity about sexuality, or more specifically to questions about condoms and their use. Not to worry! In Afghanistan, the parents knew only that condoms made terrific water balloons and had little objection to their sons' purchase of the attractive foil-wrapped packages.

GOAL: To introduce the topic of sexuality to the preteen.

Objective One: Use a youngster's questions to show readiness to learn about sexuality.

Objective Two: Understand sexuality and model composure to reduce embarrassment.

Objective Three: Discuss sexuality and reproduction in accurate terms.

Objective Four: Use familiar examples to reduce confusion about reproduction.

METHOD: Many resources help teens, parents, teachers, or ministers answer questions about sexuality. This discussion presents the reproductive systems of the male and the female in ways understandable to the preteen. It exemplifies accurate information so adults have a starting point. One develops his or her own terms and style of addressing preteen questions as comfort levels increase. For help, use the "Glossary of Reproductive Anatomy and Related Terms" on page 104.

Have the young people make a fist with either hand. Note that a fist is about the size and shape of a pear. This "pear" is the approximate size of the adult nonpregnant uterus or womb of the female. The womb is at the bottom of the abdominal cavity. A band of tissue called a broad ligament holds the uterus or womb in place.

There are three openings to the womb. The large one is the cervix or mouth of the womb and opens into the vagina. The vagina is the tube to the outside of a woman's body and accepts the penis in lovemaking called sexual intercourse. The other two openings are the fallopian tubes.

Encourage young people to use a mirror to look at their own reproductive organs. They will learn to locate parts of the body and to ask questions about taking care of themself. This is a healthy start to accepting, respecting, and protecting sexuality.

The young girl will find that the vagina is the middle opening to the outside of her body; behind it is the anus or place where solid waste leaves the body. In front of it is the urethra or tube from the bladder or bag that holds urine for liquid waste products.

When the boy looks at his body, he will see only two openings, the penis in the front and the anus in the back. Inside are a complicated set of tubes and ducts. In one area are the vas deferens where fluid called semen is added to the sperm so they can swim more easily. In the other area, urine collects in the bladder. The urethra connects the bladder to the outside of a man's body through the penis. The vas deferens joins the urethra, so the urethra is the common tube for both fluids to reach the exterior of the body.

Boys have organs on the outside of the body that hang behind the penis in a bag called the scrotum. They are called testes and are almond-shaped and almond-sized. The manufacture of sperm is in the testes. The penis has special tissues that engorge with blood to make it hard upon sexual stimulation. This allows it to enter the woman's body in sexual intercourse. Further stimulation causes ejaculation and the depositing of sperm in the vagina.

So far we have talked mostly about the reproductive system that we can see or that we can easily imagine. It will take a leap of imagination to think about a small gland in the brain called the pituitary gland. The pituitary secretes hormones that cause bodily changes in the preteen. Testosterone is the male hormone that brings about enlargement of the penis, a deepening of the voice, and hairy changes to the armpits, chest, and genital areas. Estrogen secretion in females prompts enlargement of the reproductive organs, ovulation, and adult hair growth. The breasts of a young woman begin to mature just when hormones act on the womb and periods begin. The variation in changes from person to person also represents the idea that our sexuality and our reproductive organs may differ in size and shape and still be normal.

Now the preteens will need to use their imagination as they go back to "see" the other two openings at the top of the womb of the woman. Envision taking a drinking straw and cutting it crosswise into two lengths. Then imagine a half-straw tube that comes out of each side of the womb. This tube is soft and flexible and is called a fallopian tube. At the end opposite the womb, the tube passes into the interior of the woman's body and has little filaments like tiny floating fingers waiting to grab the egg or ovum.

What is the egg? Where does it come from? And how does it get fertilized? Within reach of the free floating fallopian tubes are the woman's two almond-sized, almond-shaped reproductive organs called the ovaries. Before a girl-child is born, her ovaries contain all the eggs that will ripen and release during her lifetime. Ovulation or egg release takes place on one side for one month and alternates to the other side the following month. The egg, the largest known cell in the body of a human, is the size of the tiniest pinhead. This ovum contains one-half of the genetic material required to begin formation of the human embryo.

One ovum ripens, releases, and is swept into the fallopian tube by the filaments. If sexual intercourse takes place, there is a release from the man of millions of sperm that swim two-thirds of the way through the tube to the traveling ovum. The sperm contains the other half of the genetic building material required to produce a human. Also present is the chromosome determination of sex. Fertilization takes place when the head of one sperm unites with the egg to begin building a human being. During the previous month, the woman's body has been lining the uterus with a nutritious substance in which the embryo can implant and feed. This embryo grows into a fetus and through a nine-month gestation period to become a full-term baby. Ideally, a baby needs nine months of growth inside the womb of the mother. However, babies born as early as seven months gestational age can survive outside the womb.

If sexual intercourse to release sperm does not occur or if birth control measures block fertilization, there is no embryo to require the nutrients and safety of the prepared womb. The womb then sheds its nutritious lining and it flows through the vagina to the exterior of the woman's body as a period or menstruation. Again, the pituitary gland controls this reproductive activity by secreting a hormone. The process of preparing for fertilization repeats itself every month during the childbearing years, or for about thirty-five to forty years of a woman's life. The menstrual cycle begins in the early teen years; however, excessive athletic activity, dieting, early teen pregnancy, and heredity may alter that schedule.

QUESTIONS FOR CONSIDERATION:

1)   American youth reach puberty about two years earlier than they did a half century ago. What is the reason for this change in the rate of development?

2)   What challenges has this early development created?

3)   Is the discussion of reproductive development similar from family to family? How do we find the answer to this question?

4)   Are youngsters learning about their sexuality by the time they are two? Do they identify themselves as girls or boys?

5)   Can acceptance of one's sexuality be changed by understanding reproductive development?

6)   How would you increase your knowledge or your teen's knowledge of reproduction? What information can you find through local book stores, school libraries, parenting classes, and church programs?

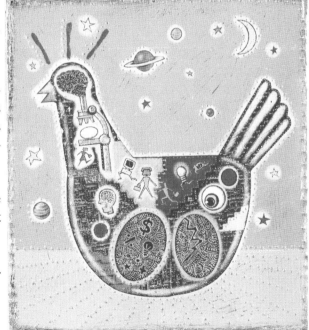

7)   What is meant by an "askable parent" and a "teachable moment?"

8)   What is the process that delays menstruation in the young person who practices excessively for athletic activities? Does this delay cause permanent damage to the reproductive system?

9)   What will happen to the manufacture and storage of sperm if clothing is too tight to permit adequate temperature changes?

10) Where is the genetic material that determines the sex of a child?

MODULE THREE
THE HEALTH QUESTIONNAIRE AND THE GENOGRAM
AS INTERVIEW TOOLS

PART ONE: THE HEALTH QUESTIONNAIRE

"Historical Perspective"

"At Highland Park, Michigan, the first Model T automobile built on a moving assembly line lurched down a ramp and came to rest in the grass under a clear sky. It was black and ungainly and stood high off the ground. Its inventor regarded it from a distance. His derby was tilted back on his head. He chewed on a piece of straw. In his left hand he held a pocket watch; he looked at his watch. Part of his genius consisted of seeming to his executives and competitors not as quick-witted as they. With his tongue he moved the straw from one corner of his mouth to the other. He looked at his watch again. Exactly six minutes after the car had rolled down the ramp, an identical car appeared at the top of the ramp, stood for a moment pointed at the cold early morning sun, then rolled down and crashed into the rear of the first one. He had been an ordinary automobile manufacturer; now he experienced a great, intense ecstasy . . . Henry Ford had caused a machine to replicate itself endlessly!"

A half-century later, Dr. Carl Djerassi walked in the gray morning stillness of Henry Ford's new Detroit. Prosperous in curiosity and determination, the young doctor pursued financial support for his ideas. That search led Djerassi to Mexico and a Central American yam that was the original source of a corticoid used in the manufacture of the birth control pill. On a mechanical assembly line on November 19, 1958, the cellophane packages of tiny white dots in a circular plastic case were first mass-produced. This tiny explosive unleashed a force greater than the liberation felt by man and his auto.

Teen pregnancy has its roots in our country's history. Two revolutionary ingredients have shaken our family foundations in such a way that we cannot turn back the clock and be the immobile, naive country folk of a century ago. The first ingredient was a mobility fostered by the industrial revolution and embodied in Henry Ford's automobile. The second ingredient was a comparable sexual emancipation embodied in "the Pill."

In the face of these revolutionary changes we maintain stability by constantly acknowledging, cultivating, and supporting family values. Within the framework of family values, individuals can contribute to our teens' comfort with adolescent changes by listening to them. So that is our starting point. A tool like the brief health questionnaire and genogram on page 25 helps one begin listening. Responses to the one-on-one interview become the main indicator of readiness for sharing and support. The interview is necessary to assess the appropriateness of group work to a teen who wants the support of his or her peers.

Angella is a slight, nervous young woman who lost her mother two years ago. Angella's family has neglected her as a small child and verbally and physically abused Angella in the recent middle school years. Her entry into high school is like a passport to independence from the family.

Other characteristics of Angella's "high school passport" include the privilege of walking with her boyfriend, Corey, whose prized possession is a red, white, and blue leather jacket with "Corvette" emblazoned on the back. Angella proudly, but secretly, tucks the phone number of a family planning agency in her hip pocket. She establishes visiting time with the school nurse and the school counselor. They can enhance Angella's self-worth and family support by listening to her and responding with a positive attitude to the few personal details Angella timidly shares.

> **GOAL: To evaluate a teen's curiosity about sexuality and his or her suitability to group work based on individual responses to the health questionnaire.**

Objective One: Increase professional awareness of teen sexuality.

Objective Two: Assess a teenager's view of sexuality to determine the risk of pregnancy.

Objective Three: Discuss family values as they affect teen pregnancy prevention.

Objective Four: Determine the risk of sexually transmitted disease.

Objective Five: Evaluate the suitability of group work to the teen interviewee.

Objective Six: Model the concept of assertiveness as it relates to reducing inappropriate sexual behaviors.

METHOD: At times when teens find it difficult to speak to their parents about sexuality, they seek the help of peers, teachers, counselors, health care professionals, and ministers for answers. Indirect questions or requests disguise their curiosity because most teenagers are embarrassed to ask directly about sexual concerns. Fear of an untimely pregnancy is the most frank sexual matter bringing teens to adults. The health questionnaire and genogram found on page 25 is an organized, yet nonthreatening, way to record teen visits. Through the progress made at these appointments one can also determine whether group work will help the young person.

The health questionnaire is an effective interview tool for a variety of reasons. First, it is brief and interactive to avoid loss of the teen's attention. Second, combined with the genogram, it asks the key questions that clarify and establish accuracy of the young person's answers. Last, it helps to decide whether the teen is ready for group work.

Questions one and two document demographic and baseline data. Question three about family health increases a teen's awareness of factors affecting sexuality, abstinence, and birth control. It also asks for his or her perspective of teen pregnancy and sexually transmitted disease. Question three helps the professional begin building a plan of care.

Succeeding parts of the health questionnaire become more personal; for example, questions four through seven ask directly about abstinence, sexual activity, and birth control. These questions also help the teen recognize and use help that will prevent conception. Sometimes it feels less personal to the teen when he or she talks to other persons before approaching parents. Professionals support family or guardian involvement and they work toward the time and circumstances that make it easier for a teen to talk to their parents or guardians. For that reason, the words "contract date" or "contract to talk to parents" is a reminder of that need for parental involvement.

Questions eight through ten are for teens who are sexually active. It enables the adolescent and the professional to talk about disease risks encountered with sexual activity and to curb the idea that it is "cool" to have multiple partners in sexual relationships. Answers to the questions introduce good health care if a sexually transmitted disease is present.

The health questionnaire is an effective tool for men and women. Corey, Angella's boyfriend, is a teen whose answers in one-on-one conversations with adults are introspective. His teachers consider Corey a capable student because he tries to analyze and support the answers that are correct in his judgment. When we came to one of the last questions of the health questionnaire, "Have you ever forced or been forced to have intercourse?" Corey answered indignantly, "Yes, that's why Angella might be pregnant; I'm not the first guy to get loaded and screw on a dare! Get real!" This honest answer gave a new meaning to "forced to have intercourse." In his view, Corey was "forced" by his friends to save face by getting drunk and fulfilling a dare. Angella's view was that she was willing to have intercourse. These differences in viewing sexuality make the health questionnaire so important when reaching and teaching teenagers.

Because fear of teen pregnancy is the most common reproductive concern requiring professional support, it calls for further discussion. Several tools measure pregnancy. The calendar and timing of sexual activity establish the possibility of conception. A blood test will accurately show pregnancy because specific hormone levels rise in the blood within ten days of conception. If an interval of forty-five days exists between the last menstrual period and the date of testing, a less costly urine test is accurate for pregnancy determination. The urine must be collected from the first morning void because that is when human chorionic gonadotropic hormone, HCG, the indicator of pregnancy, is high enough for accurate pregnancy testing.

If a pregnancy test is positive, decisions need to be made. Keeping the child, open or closed adoption, or abortion become important decisions to discuss. Module Sixteen, entitled, "Other Pregnancy Outcomes" presents different options. Resolving the outcome of a teen pregnancy is the choice of the pregnant teen, her partner, and her family. Professionals play an educational and a supporting role in the discussion. They acknowledge and accept the decision of the teens and their families.

Adolescents trust people easily. A person working with a teen is in a confidential relationship; that confidentiality extends to demographic details as well. A counselor shares information only by written permission of the teen. This, by law, includes disclosure to parents. However, "Objective Three" of this module shows the importance of fostering healthy teen-parent relationships as a regular part of counseling. The contract language to encourage parental involvement has been discussed, even most ultra-independent teens or teens living in group homes ultimately want and need the support and attention of their parents.

Discussions about family values and relationships lay the groundwork for the trust-building of group process. The completed health questionnaire helps a facilitator decide if group work is appropriate to the needs of the teen without making that adolescent feel abnormal or unique. The teen's desire to become part of a group and the parental or guardian permission to do group work are the remaining decisions to be made. No teen may join a support group without parental or guardian consent. In schools, establish this condition as a part of school policy so that it applies to students living on their own or students over eighteen years of age. A teen who is severely traumatized or has a diagnosed psychotic problem is more skillfully served through indvidual counseling sessions with an experienced practitioner.

Up to this point we have not addressed assertiveness; Module Seven is devoted to this topic. The modeling of assertive behavior by parents and professionals as they deal with teen questions is a concrete and healthy way to begin teaching assertiveness. One also introduces, demonstrates, and rehearses assertiveness by the way activities are presented as group work progresses.

To close our discussion we can summarize the areas of concern addressed by the health questionnaire; they are: 1) raising awareness and identifying resources to help prevent teen pregnancy in the first place, 2) guiding a teen to appropriate sources of help for sexual concerns, 3) using the questionnaire to build a prevention-centered care plan, 4) modeling assertiveness to reduce inappropriate sexual behaviors, 5) extending proper reproductive health care and information about sexually transmitted disease such as herpes, chlamydia, HIV/AIDS, hepatitis B, gonorrhea, venereal warts, or syphilis, 6) establishing legal and personal counseling contacts when such issues as date or statutory rape are involved, and 7) using the health questionnaire to track general statistics and outcomes to build a continuing program of prevention.

QUESTIONS FOR CONSIDERATION:

1)   Does your community provide adequate resources in response to teen curiosity about their sexuality? What resources are available?

2)   Is sexuality education solely the responsibility of a parent? Informally interview a teenager, a doctor, a lawyer, a businessperson, a minister, and a teacher about their view of responsibility to the reproductive health of teens.

3)   Is disclosure of demographic data a confidential concern?

4)   When investigating materials, how important is information on sexual abstinence? What programs offer information on abstinence? Refer to the "Resource Guide" on page 115.

5)   This module alludes to the value of pregnancy testing; it does not include a discussion about home pregnancy tests. Investigate home pregnancy tests on the market and evaluate their accuracy.

6)   Family health problems contribute to risk factors in teen sexuality; what are some health concerns that might surface during the interview?

7)   Should a school staff member send a pregnant teen from school to other agencies without parental or guardian permission?

8)   Why is the subject of HIV/AIDS a part of the health questionnaire?

9)   Find and list current hotline available for anonymously answering teen questions on HIV/AIDS and other sexually transmitted diseases. Watch and listen for public service announcements on television and radio.

10) Brochures about HIV/AIDS and other sexually transmitted disease are not provided with this guide book. Investigate the availability of information from local or state resources; how can one help provide information brochures on sexual health and related issues to adolescents?

PART TWO: THE GENOGRAM

"Breaking The Cycle"

I see Angella in my office for the third time. She comes rubbing her jaw and exclaiming about the pain caused by her new braces. "Okay," I reply. "You need written permission from your mother or the doctor to take a pain reliever." "I don't have a mom," she answers bitterly, with a defensive head toss that is just a bit too slow to hide the tears that silently slip down her cheeks and spread in dark pools on her red shirt. "She died two years ago. Anyway it doesn't matter. This is just the worst day of my life!"

"I am sorry," I respond. In reality, I have known of Angella's loss, but her feelings are not real to me until that moment. She relates how difficult it is making the choice to see someone about her fear. Angella has not had her period in more than nine weeks and is afraid that she is pregnant. We look at a calendar and explore the possibility of a pregnancy by what dates intercourse took place. Often teens do not have regular cycles. Even with regular cycles, a woman may become pregnant at any time of the month unless abstinence or birth control mechanisms control fertilization.

One also questions what methods of avoiding pregnancy Angella and Corey understand and use. Angella replies, "We use condoms when we have money and time to buy them, but we don't do *it* that often so I didn't think we would have a baby. Now I'm scared!"

Angella's response naturally prompts a question about the availability of immediate family support. Angella replies, "My aunt who is now my mother is good support, but I *won't* tell her anything unless I'm pregnant!" Angella agrees to ask her boyfriend, Corey, if he is willing to stop and chat. We establish a tentative appointment. After some encouraging, Corey and Angella are willing to go to Planned Parenthood for counseling and pregnancy testing after school.

One will notice that, officially or unofficially, items from the health questionnaire are introduced. However, the genogram becomes the tool to help Angella and Corey see the importance of their families for support. The genogram graphically strengthens the idea of family connections. The use of the genogram in a pregnancy prevention program is an outgrowth of a trend in our society to reexamine family roots and the genealogy that gives us individual distinction. Family and given names provide simple reinforcement of an individual's heritage. The genogram helps discover such connections. Further, helping a teen relate to their family tree, supports pride in their heritage. It is another concrete way to promote the self-worth of an adolescent.

When an adolescent visits on a regular basis, using the genogram is helpful to remember the teen's immediate and extended family. A glance at this visual aid tells the counselor or the health care professional what motivation beyond the presenting situation may be affecting the teen. Furthermore, a teen enjoys the mutual approach of this graphic way to see family connections. Concerns are put in a family context and can be examined for patterns that influence day-to-day living. The responsibility of pregnancy prevention rests squarely on a teen's shoulders, but the connection with support shows he or she is not alone.

Taking ownership of risky behaviors and establishing relationships with parents and helping professionals are two specific steps that a teen can take to prevent teen pregnancy.

Taking ownership of risky behaviors and establishing relationships with parents and helping professionals are two specific steps that a teen can take to prevent teen pregnancy. About two-thirds of the teens who "stress out" over their sexually active, risk-taking behaviors have their period after they talk to someone. As it happened, Angella and Corey were not pregnant. The genogram helps the health care professional support Angella and Corey as they come to visit in subsequent months. This couple and their friends feel that attention to their questions about sexuality contributes to their resolve to delay pregnancy. In support groups as well, continued discussion, documentation, support, and hugs become invaluable ingredients for preventing first and subsequent pregnancies.

GOAL: To understand the contribution heritage makes to promoting or breaking the cycle of teen pregnancy.

Objective One: Define the genogram or family heritage diagram.

Objective Two: Understand the significance of family positions and family expectations.

Objective Three: Diagram the family heritage by using symbols.

Objective Four: Use the genogram to portray family values and relationships in an individual setting and then in a confidential group setting.

METHOD: Identity is important to self-realization; maintain a personal bond by addressing a person by their name. Family heritage and spirituality are also part of a person's singularity and build one's unique identity. Family roles are a part of identity. Acknowledging a teen's role within the family is affirming to that adolescent. Discussing family origins and values help a teen identify family expectations. These expectations play a major role in the teen's view of sexuality and decisions to delay pregnancy.

Author Sharon Wegscheider-Cruse writes about family relationships and systems. The terms she uses were first coined to describe the roles of the chemically dependent person and the codependent family. The chemically dependent person's actions and attitudes in response to chemical abuse undermine healthy relationships within a family. The "chief enabler" covers, denies, or generally hides the family problems that begin to develop in response to the chemical abuse. The enabler, usually the spouse, is ever-vigilant and controlling in order to preserve family balance. In that reactive stance he relegates himself to family duties and influence that deny selfhood and self-love. If the family situation is not remedied, all family members develop rigid roles that maintain family homeostasis.

The preceding description may apply to a family where teen pregnancy is a symptom of imbalance and family dysfunction. In the enmeshed family of that pregnant teen, roles are rigid. When a family member finds a place for himself, he clings to that role because it is his identity. The "hero" is usually the oldest child who is the standard bearer and proclaims family equilibrium to the outside world by showing how positive, capable, and loveable the family is. The "scapegoat" acts out troubles and stands as a reactionary to the goodness of the "hero." He says, "There's no way my life is going to be as boring and predictable as my sister's; I want lots of friends, places to go, and things to do." This stance often leads to risk-taking behavior that is hidden and challenging to parents and their ability to cope with adolescent changes.

The "lost child" is the child who fades into anonymity and does not expect to get his or her needs met. The "mascot" feigns a light heart because the gravity of the family situation needs comic relief. Both the "lost child" and the "mascot" function to relieve the anxieties of the family system. Any one of the young people who display the characteristics of a dysfunctional family may be vulnerable to early pregnancy. Discuss family roles and boundaries while building the genogram. Here is the way to proceed.

First, by reading Angella's health questionnaire and genogram handout found on page 26, one will note from the demographic and health data that she is an average student with a moderate number of school absences. Angella has a low, regular pulse and blood pressure that is normal to her age group. She is slight in body size for her height but is not underweight according to standard actuarial height and weight graphs. Her vision is corrected by contacts and her hearing is good by report and ability to hear a conversation. Angella wears braces for dental correction.

All family health concerns have a bearing on pregnancy, but the continued use of medication such as "pain-killers" and proventil or other asthma and allergy medications could have a teratogenic effect on a fetus. It is noted that use of medications was continued over the nine-week period when there was the possibility of pregnancy. One will also note that clotting problems, toxemia, and thyroid problems among the women of Angella's family circle affect prenatal growth.

Continue to the space at the bottom of the form; the interviewer or interviewee draw the genogram or family tree. A genogram is simply a line drawing of the family system. Drawing the family tree becomes a nonthreatening, imaginative way to help a teenager recount the significance of family health and family connections. Teens, both male and female, learn that healthy family patterns or the lack of them influence their view of sexuality.

The diagram also shows relationships of family members across different generations. The lines join Angella, the key person, to her immediate family and then to the extended family to create three strata or generations. If Angella had been pregnant, four strata would have shaped her family tree at this time in her life. Some diagrams or genograms are complex; however, using a minimum of symbols for simplicity and clarity is effective, see "Genogram Symbols" on page 24. There are a few basic signs used in genograms. However, one may make up his own symbols if he chooses. Protect confidentiality of the teen and store the genogram in a locked file or give the teen a choice about keeping this personal written information.

Now examine Angella's genogram at the bottom of page 26. Note the standard symbols used in diagraming Angella's family. The square symbolizes a living male and the circle symbolizes a living female. The age of the person is represented by a number within the square or circle. If a famly member has died, a slash through the square or circle indicates death and the number within the circle is the age at the time of death. The person of prime importance is the star person and is represented by lines or spokes circling the main character around whom the family genogram is built.

Relationships are shown by various lines. For example a solid line between a square and a circle shows marriage, a broken line between a man and a woman shows a joining relationship but not a marriage. A single slash on a marriage line shows a separation; a double slash indicates divorce. A single slash on a relationship line shows that the partners are no longer together.

We will study the strata of Angella's genogram. The line of the middle stratum shows a marriage that ended in divorce. The man is presently thirty-three years old and is Angella's father. Angella's mother is deceased and died at thirty-one. They had three children as indicated by the line that extends downward to a male symbol of twelve, a female symbol of fourteen, and the star person of Angella, aged sixteen, around whom the heritage circle is built.

On the remaining heritage lines to the left and to the right of Angella's parents are the siblings of her thirty-three year old father and her deceased mother. Angella does not know a great deal about her father. She has not seen him for many years. Angella only knows that he has one brother who is possibly still alive and was known as "an alcoholic." She does not know her paternal grandparents except that her grandmother is "about fifty" and lives in Chicago.

Angella's genogram confirms strong ties to her mother's family. Angella's maternal grandparents are an integral part of her life and have always been the ones to give her loving support. Her grandfather is fifty-three and in good health with a job for the state highway department. Her grandmother does not work because "she has high blood pressure." She is fifty-one years old and weighs about "two hundred and fifty pounds."

Look at the family pattern of teen pregnancy. Notice that on both sides of Angella's genealogy her grandmothers became mothers at an early age. One grandmother had a child at fourteen years of age; the other had her first child at seventeen. If these patterns are not acknowledged by discussion, a teen will not realize that there may be an unspoken acceptance or expectation of teen pregnancy in the family heritage circle.   These details could contribute to Angella's expectations of herself. Angella may not consciously realize that she has the right to make decisions about childbearing for herself. And that she has the right to break the cycle with tools that increase decision-making and problem-solving.

As we move back to the middle stratum of the genogram, we see that Angella has an aunt and uncle who are thirty-five and thirty-seven, respectively. Her aunt's heritage line to the thirty-four-year-old male indicates a marriage that is still intact. Angella's uncle by marriage and her maternal uncle own a trucking service together. Angella's aunt is the person who has unofficially adopted Angella and her siblings. As Angella's genogram and questionnaire relate, her "aunt-mother" had several miscarriages before conceiving a single son who is ten years old. Angella was the product of a teen pregnancy when Angella's mother was seventeen years old.

Angella has fair grades, although she would rather stay home than attend school. She timidly shares that she misses her mother a lot and has never told anyone how much she wants to leave her aunt's household and "be on her own." She denies any health problems and does not smoke. Angella says she has been known to drink at parties, and has been drunk at least twice in the last nine weeks. Angella adds that she would be happy if she were pregnant, but she hopes she isn't.

Angella has a sister who is fourteen and a model student in school. This is exemplified by good grades, good school attendance, and competitive sports accomplishments. In studying this genogram one might look at the rigidity or fluidity of the roles that the children in this family display. Angella relates "my brother is often gone from home even though he is only twelve." She continues, "He usually hangs out with his friends and smokes; he does not like school and the doctor says he is 'hyperactive.'" Angella thinks her brother is now taking a medication to "help him keep still."

Now look at Corey's genogram on page 27. It is blank. How are the following paragraphs of details used to build Corey's questionnaire and genogram? Corey is the sixteen-year-old star person around whom his genogram is transcribed. He has an eighteen-year-old sister who "works at J.C.Penney and buys her own clothes." Corey's sister has a "bad heart and is babied" by Corey's thirty-five-year-old mother. Corey has never known his father, although he lives in the same town as Corey. Corey feels "left alone" by this man who never married his mother. Corey's step-father acts like a dad and is one year older than Corey's mother. Corey does not know much about his natural father's parents except that Corey's mother heard from that side of the family when the grandmother died of a stroke. Corey believes that his grandfather is in his early sixties and that he has a paternal aunt who is about the same age as his mother, that is, about thirty-five. Corey sometimes feels that he should be "babied" too because his stomach "feels like it has an ulcer." The fear of pregnancy has made Corey "feel like vomiting and running away."

Corey says, "My grandparents are there for me." He has been helping his grandfather who is in his middle fifties and had a foot removed because "it had gangrene after a hunting accident." His grandmother is "just beyond turning fifty" and never leaves the house. Corey's mother has been pregnant twice in the last few years but has lost the babies. Note that the strata of Corey's genogram show a pattern of teen pregnancy.

Corey's mother is a "heavy smoker and a drinker." She is a very "good person" and pays Corey when he gets on the honor roll. Corey is proud of his quick wit and his good academic standing. He has an uncle who is "is a druggie" and Corey says, "I hate to admit that the guy is my uncle." Corey thinks he has about five other aunts and uncles. Corey rarely sees them and does not know their names.

Collecting the preceding data illustrates the use of a genogram for social and health information. The genogram can show birth order, health problems, early pregnancies, drug abuse, and belief systems of the extended family. Professionals other than the health care providers can construct a genogram that speaks to different points of need. For example, teachers and ministers could use the concept of a genogram in their classroom or in their ministry. These extensions of the genogram are dealt with in successive modules.

The simplicity of collecting data via a genogram is evident. This one-page information key is used to refresh one's memory and to add new details as they become important to the health and welfare of a teenager. In all situations, information shared by a person is confidential and is offered for safe-keeping to the individual to whom the genogram belongs. At no time is a young person forced or coerced to answer a health questionnaire or genogram; he or she may stop the process at any time. No information may be shared except by written permission of the teenager. All confidential materials are kept in a locked file. A computer is not used because a computerized record cannot be stored with assurance of strict confidentiality.

Genogram Symbols

[ ] - square represents male

O   - circle represents female

/   - to cover a square or circle shows person has died
number within the square or circle indicates age at which deceased died

[7] - number inside square or circle indicates age

[[]] - star or key person or presenting student has a double-line circle or square

[ ]--------O- solid line between the square and the circle shows marriage

[ ]- - - - -O- broken line between the square and the circle shows joining but not a marriage

[ ]---\----O- a single slash on a marriage line indicates separation

[ ]---\\---O- a double slash on a marriage line indicates divorce

[ ]- -\- - -O- a single slash on a joining line indicates that the couple are no longer together

Health Questionnaire and Genogram

Health Questionnaire

This is a confidential questionnaire to be done with a health professional. If you do not feel comfortable answering a question, a "pass" response is okay. Use the reverse side of the questionnaire for expanded answers.

1. General Data: initials _____ date_____ age_____ sex_____ grades_____attendance_____
2. Health Data: vision____ hearing____ blood pressure____ pulse____ height____weight____
3. Do you or your close family members have any of the following health problems?

    a. cancer____   infections____   seizures____
        diabetes____   clotting problems____   medications____
        asthma____   miscarriages____   substance abuse____
        heart disease____   premature births____   operations____

    b. Do you or does anyone in your family have a handicap?____ disorder? ____
    disability?____ emotional problem?____

4. (Young women) How often are your periods?____ amount?____ duration?____
    problems?____
5. Are you sexually active?____ one partner?____
6. Do you and/or your partner use birth control?____ kind used?____ starting date____
    problems?____
7. Have you ever thought you were pregnant?____ positive or negative test?____
8. Are you able to talk to your parents about dating?____ birth control?____ pregnancy?____
    STDs____ HIV/AIDS?____ contract date ____
9. Have you ever had pain when you pass water?____ Have you had an infection of the
    vagina?____ the penis?____
10. Have you ever been forced to have intercourse?____

Genogram: Health, Heritage, Spirituality

Angella's Health Questionnaire and Genogram

Health Questionnaire

This is a confidential questionnaire to be done with a health professional. If you do not feel comfortable answering a question, a "pass" response is okay. Use the reverse side of the questionnaire for expanded answers.

1. General Data: initials **A.T.** date **4/16/96** age **16** sex **♀** grades **2.7 gpa** attendance **4 absences 2d sem.**
2. Health Data: vision **p** hearing **p** blood pressure **106/64** pulse **68** height **5'8"** weight **154 lbs.**
3. Do you or your close family members have any of the following health problems?
   a. cancer **+ mother deceased - breast cancer**   infections **θ**   seizures **θ**
   diabetes **θ**   clotting problems **+ maternal gmother**   medications **+ mother on thyroid**
   asthma **+ self - uses proventil**   miscarriages **θ**   substance abuse **paternal gfather, uncle**
   heart disease **θ**   premature births **+ aunt**   operations **+ thyroidectomy**
   b. Do you or does anyone in your family have a handicap? **θ**   disorder? **+ brother, learning dis.**
   disability? **θ**   emotional problem? **+ self - misses mother**
4. (Young women) How often are your periods? **month** amount? **mod.** duration? **4-5 days** problems? **occasional cramps, irregularity**
5. Are you sexually active? **+**   one partner? **+**
6. Do you and/or your partner use birth control? **+**   kind used? **condoms** starting date **≅ 2/1/96** problems? **sometimes don't use birth control**
7. Have you ever thought you were pregnant? **+**   positive or negative test? **? fear due to 2 missed periods**
8. Are you able to talk to your parents about dating? **+**   birth control? **θ**   pregnancy? **θ** STDs? **θ**   HIV/AIDS? **θ**   contract date? **by 5/15/96**
9. Have you ever had pain when you pass water? **θ**   Have you had an infection of the vagina? **θ**   the penis? **N/A**
10. Have you ever been forced to have intercourse? **θ**

Genogram: Health, Heritage, Spirituality

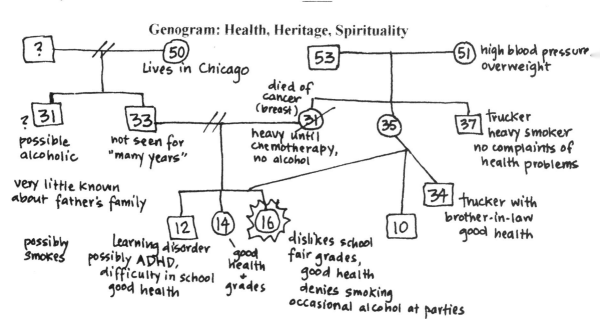

Corey's Health Questionnaire and Genogram

Health Questionnaire

This is a confidential questionnaire to be done with a health professional. If you do not feel comfortable answering a question, a "pass" response is okay. Use the reverse side of the questionnaire for expanded answers.

1. General Data: initials_____ date_____ age_____ sex_____ grades_____ attendance_____
2. Health Data: vision____ hearing____ blood pressure____ pulse____ height____weight____
3. Have you or any of your close family members had any of the following health problems?
   a. cancer____   infections____   seizures____
       diabetes____   clotting problems____   medications____
       asthma____   miscarriages____   substance abuse____
       heart disease____   premature births____   operations____
   b. Do you or does anyone in your family have a handicap?____ disorder?____ disability?____ emotional problem?____
4. (Young women) How often are your periods?____ amount?____ duration?____ problems?____
5. Are you sexually active?____ one partner?____
6. Do you and/or your partner use birth control?____ kind used?____ starting date____ problems?____
7. Have you ever thought you were pregnant?____ positive or negative test?____
8. Are you able to talk to your parents about dating?____ birth control?____ pregnancy?____

   STDs____ HIV/AIDS?____ contract date ____
9. Have you ever had pain when you pass water?____ Have you had an infection of the vagina?____ the penis?____
10. Have you ever been forced to have intercourse?____

Genogram: Health, Heritage, Spirituality

QUESTIONS FOR CONSIDERATION:

1)   What significance does the diagnosed breast cancer of a sixty-year-old woman have to the reproductive health of her granddaughter?

2)   What is the health professional's responsibility if one discusses and records a genetic disorder and no one outside the immediate family is aware of it?

3)   Explain the connection between the family expectations of a pregnant teen and her motivation to care for a child.   Consider such issues as open or closed adoption, availability of child care, pregnancy termination, graduation from high school, vocational school, or college, and grief concerns of the pregnant teen.

4)   Is silence about a teen's decision regarding pregnancy prevention affirming or not?

5)   According to John Bradshaw and Sharon Wegscheider-Cruse, specialists in chemical dependency counseling, ordinal birth order makes a difference in family expectations of a child. What are the names given to the different positions and what do they mean?

6)   Study Angella's completed health questionnaire and genogram as shown on page 26. Practice completing Corey's questionnaire and genogram on page 27 from the information on page 23.

7)   Complete a genogram by drawing your family heritage.

8)   In completing your own genogram, was a perspective of teen sexuality expressed? Were branches of your family practicing abstinence; did others experience teen pregnancy?

9)   Was there coincidence of alcohol abuse and teen pregnancy?

10) Do you have any examples of "breaking the cycle" in your extended family background? How is that cycle of teen pregnancy broken?

MODULE FOUR
GROUP GROUND RULES

"In Case of Confidentiality"

Case law from the annals of the California Supreme Court describes *Tarasoff versus the Regents of the University of California*, a decision that has had unique influence on counselor/client confidentiality. In the Tarasoff case, the counselor, Moore, a psychologist working for the Student Health Service on the Berkeley campus was counseling, Poddar. Moore believed Poddar had the potential to kill his intended victim, Tarasoff. The counselor reported Poddar's homicidal ideation to the campus police.

The police questioned Poddar and they dismissed him as a rational person and not a danger to Tarasoff. However, neither Moore nor the police informed Tarasoff that Poddar had said he would kill her. Poddar did kill Tarasoff and Tarasoff's parents sued the Regents of the University of California, maintaining that their daughter had the right to know that her life was in jeopardy and should have been warned so that she could protect herself. The final decision agreed with the parent's declaration of the psychologist's and police officers' negligence to communicate a potential danger to their daughter.

Tarasoff versus the Regents of the University of California redefined the counselor/client relationship. The 1976 California Supreme Court decision regarding Tarasoff set a precedent allowing physicians, coun-

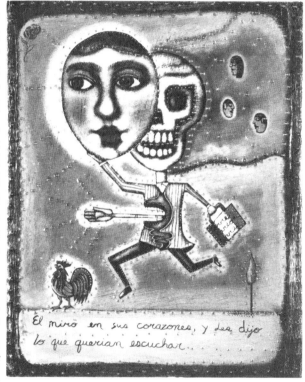

El miró en sus corazones, y les dijo lo que querían escuchar...

selors, psychologists, or other similar care givers the right to compromise client confidentiality to protect a suicidal patient or client from himself or to safeguard an intended victim of homicide from the alleged perpetrator.

GOAL: To help teen participants learn, establish, and model fair play and appropriate group ground rules.

Objective One: Define and describe the basic parameters of group work.

Objective Two: Define boundaries of confidentiality.

Objective Three: Foster honesty by requiring teens to: 1) inform their parent or guardian, in writing, of participation in the group, 2) be responsible for homework that is missed due to group work, and 3) say "goodbye" if a teen decides to leave the group.

Objective Four: Affirm participants by recognizing, discussing, and reducing put-downs.

Objective Five: Recognize that we do not make decisions for other people; we choose to or not to support the decisions they make for themselves.

Objective Six: Model appropriate dress and affection within the group.

METHOD: Ice breakers, introductions, and group ground rules are the activities for the opening sessions of work with teens. Group work takes many forms. It may be open or closed; it may meet weekly or biweekly; it may include men and women; or it may or may not augment individual counseling sessions. Basic needs of the group will determine the direction of the work.

Beside making decisions about ground rules, it is necessary to present general information about expectations and changes with each new stage of group work. We will discuss ground rules within the context of group phase one. The first phase of group process is building parallel relationships, or *forming*. The goal of this phase is to begin building trust of one another so that group members have a working model to examine. This stage culminates in affirming members about what they believe they see and feel.

How does one begin establishing trust? First, ground rules of operation are necessary. These rules, as outlined on page 32, are established at the first meeting of the group and represent a written agreement validating boundaries. Discussing rules together means communicating on a safe and basic level. This is the beginning of relationships that are not threatening to group members. These relationships also encourage individual attendance on a committed basis. Allowing a person to make mistakes is a manner of empowering him or her. Group ownership belongs to its teen members when they establish their own rules. They may make mistakes about the boundaries they choose. The teens more fully understand these mistakes if they have ownership of their work and feel the consequences of ill-defined

Group members learn trust and how to communicate without guilt if they are repeatedly affirmed and not chastised for expressing feelings.

boundaries. A key role of the counselor is to keep communication "safe."   Group members learn trust and how to communicate without guilt if they are repeatedly affirmed and not chastised for expressing feelings.

Phase two, or the inclusion phase, reflects a major commitment to establishing unconditional acceptance of each group member. Phase two is called *norming.* New members carefully hide their concerns and do not want to hurt anyone's feelings. What an adolescent has done in the past is not the issue. Any feeling shared is affirmed and investigated; it is not judged by a label of "good" or "bad."

Roles of leadership are noted about four meetings into group work; other roles will not assert themselves until the group process encourages deeper adolescent commitment to honest sharing. Group meetings in phase three may result in *storming,* or disagreement, because honesty permits presenting and acknowledging a variety of different and even opposing points of view. Establishing the mutuality of stage three begins with exercises of the mandala or sharing of one's spiritual core. Trusting enough to show honest feelings is the most important outcome of empowerment and is the hallmark of personal growth through group work.

Stage four is that of closure or *conforming.* Planning for the future takes place with different intensity for each group member. A facilitator's obligation is to validate these different feelings and guard that enough time is given to a member who needs help separating from the group.

In individual or group counseling, preserving confidentiality is an important right of the participants. The ground rules clearly state that "everything we say in group, stays in group." The students who are present when the group is established at the beginning of a school year either discuss and adopt the standing ground rules of the previous year's group or establish limits of their own.

Group decisions about confidentiality are written in a variety of ways. The rules need to state clearly when and why confidentiality may need to be compromised. Look at the example of "Group Ground Rules" on page 32. Number three under confidentiality states, "Life threatening gestures require the decision of the facilitator."   At the beginning of group work, members decide that indicators about suicidal gestures will be dealt with and privately negotiated outside of the group to the benefit of the person in danger. "Mandatory reporting of child abuse or neglect," means that suspected or documented child abuse or neglect must be reported to authorized child care advocates.

When the introductory phase of a group comes to a close, each member will understand their commitment to the confidential nature of group sharing. A member will need to choose a witness as they sign the commitment to confidentiality and limits as found in the ground rules.

Group Ground Rules

CONFIDENTIALITY.

    1. What is said in the room is to stay here.

    2. No gossiping.

    3. Life threatening gestures require decision of the facilitator.

APPROPRIATE DRESS AND AFFECTION IN GROUP.

NO PUT-DOWNS ANYWHERE.

A "PASS" RESPONSE IS OKAY.

IF ONE DECIDES TO LEAVE THE GROUP, OFFICIAL APPEARANCE TO SAY GOODBYE IS NECESSARY.

PARENT KNOWLEDGE OF TEEN PARTICIPATION IN GROUP.

ALL HOMEWORK MISSED NEEDS TO BE MADE UP.

SUPPORT EACH OTHER'S DECISIONS REGARDING DECISIONS.

MANDATORY REPORTING OF SUSPECTED CHILD ABUSE.

First Names and Phone Numbers of Group Participants for Sharing:

I agree with and will abide by the Group Ground Rules.

Name:_____   Date: _____

Witness: _____   Date: _____

QUESTIONS FOR CONSIDERATION:

1)   Discuss problems that develop if parental permission is not a requisite to joining a group that focuses on the management of teen sexuality.

2)   Should males and females attend the same group if teen sexuality is the topic of discussion; should teen mothers and fathers participate in the same group?

3)   What points need discussion when establishing guidelines for "appropriate behavior, dress, and affection" within a teen group?

4)   Why are the recognition, discussion, and reduction of put-downs affirming to group participants?

5)   How would you handle a continual "pass" response from the same member?

6)   Discuss trust. Which group characteristics show an escalating trust level?

7)   How and why does gossip undermine group trust levels and what are the characteristics of a group where trust is de-escalating?

8)   What would a group facilitator do about the boundaries of confidentiality if he or she knew that a pregnant teen were neglecting his or her child?

9)   What would the counselor do if a teen was in danger of committing suicide?

10) What type of support is appropriate to the teen who chooses abortion? Discuss your answer.

* The questions for consideration at the end of Module Four, "Group Ground Rules" make one aware of the diverse concerns when facilitating group work. Read and consider them at the end of Module Four, then return to answer them after reading Modules Five through Eighteen.

MODULE FIVE
COOKIE BAKE AND CAREER NIGHT

"For The Love Of Agape"

"There is no safe investment," C.S.Lewis shares in his book, *The Four Loves*. "To love at all is to be vulnerable. Love anything, and your heart will certainly be wrung and possibly be broken. If you want to make sure of keeping it intact, you must give your heart to no one, not even an animal."

"Wrap it carefully round with hobbies and little luxuries; avoid all entanglements; lock it safe in the casket of your own selfishness. But in that casket - safe, dark, motionless, airless - it will change. It will not be broken; it will become unbreakable, impenetrable." Lewis writes further, "I believe that the most lawless and inordinate loves are less contrary to God's will than a self-invited and self-protective lovelessness." C.S. Lewis calls an intense unconditional interest and love of others "agape love." Often teens who are vulnerable to unintended pregnancy do not realize that love of and interest in another person, even of the opposite sex, can exist without exploiting erotic feelings.

Dr. Bailey Molineux, a family therapist, puts it well in a piece called "The Four Types of Love" from *The Good Enough Family.* He writes, "In examining relations, therapists make a distinction between healthy and unhealthy, addictive love. Ideally, in a healthy loving relationship, many, but not all of our psychological needs are met by our spouse. We know we are special to another human being. As a result of that love, we feel better about our lives and ourselves."

Dr. Molineux continues, "The irony of the difference between healthy and unhealthy love is that unhealthy love feels stronger than healthy love. The person has such a desperate need for approval that whatever scraps of love he or she occasionally receives are experienced as wonderful. The person is on a roller-coaster ride of passion and pain, acceptance and rejection, which keeps him or her hooked in an addictive relationship."

Wrapping one's heart up so it cannot be broken is evident in the struggles, avoidance, and gestures teens demonstrate at various times in their growth to adulthood or early parenthood. Baking cookies and making plans for the future seem impractical and distant at a time when immediate responsibilities are all-consuming. Yet it is the homeliness of cookies and careers that keep us in touch with reality. They symbolize the hope, the goodness of day to day living, and the value of spouses, family members, true friends, and constant companions whose eyes reflect acceptance of us just the way we are.

Cookie Bake and Career Night are big steps. They mark the breaking away from safe and predictable messages and the beginning of sincere corporate sharing.

GOAL: To use the common goals of career plans and social interests to form group bonds.

Objective One: Form social bonds.

Objective Two: Plan and organize a group event outside the safety of the common meeting place and agenda.

Objective Three: Bake cookies as a refreshment for Career Night or a similar event.

Objective Four: Create a Career Night atmosphere where teens and families who have common concerns acquaint themselves with the career counselor, the career center, and material available for graduation, vocational success and/or college careers.

METHOD: We hold Cookie Bake and Career Night on two consecutive evenings when the group is developing a spirit of comradery. For the first evening, planning and ingredients for baking are a contribution of each group member. A teen volunteers his home for the activity.

On the second night, the Career Center is open during evening hours to bring teens and their families together to discuss graduation and career goals. The career counselor is introduced and he or she presents information about vocational and career opportunities.

The Cookie Bake and Career Night are examples of social events that are effective for building trust and support in any teen group which includes sexuality and the prevention of teen pregnancy as part of their agenda. Examples are teen institutes and insight groups for the reduction of substance abuse, church groups, support groups for eating disorders, and teen pregnancy and parenting groups preventing a second pregnancy.

Cookie Bake and Career Night or similar events promote group bonding. Meeting under new circumstances represents leaving one's safety zone. To some teens this is very easy, yet to others, it is a challenge that requires courage that is supported because group members are acquainted with one another.

QUESTIONS FOR CONSIDERATION:

1) Collect favorite cookie recipes for sharing.

2) Collect and share favorite inspirational stories and poems.

3) What community organizations and agencies beside the school provide vocational education and job opportunities for teens?

4) Do these same agencies have an integrated program that provides help to the college bound student?

5) When one investigates career and counseling centers, note whether brochures and information are available on teen sexuality and pregnancy prevention. Is it appropriate to have this information available? Why or why not?

6) Look at Erikson's stages of development on page 46. The preteen years are called the age of "industry versus inferiority" and the major goal of healthy preteen development is "to become absorbed in tasks and productive pursuits." How does your community use this information to maximize preteen interest in their future and prevent teen pregnancy?

7) Is it important that pregnant and parenting teens complete high school and have opportunity for skilled jobs and college?

8) If a family with a pregnant teen moves to the community, where could they go for teen job and career training?

9) How is the school curriculum built to support the career and job needs of pregnant and parenting students?

10) When is it appropriate to invite teens with their babies to school? List the pros and cons of this opportunity.

MODULE SIX
USING THE MANDALA

"Collect"

God comes forth in the sign of the Arousing.
    He brings all things to completion in the sign of the Gentle.
    He causes creatures to perceive each other in the sign of the Light.
    He causes them to serve one another in the sign of the Receptive.
    He gives them joy in the sign of the Joyous.
    He battles in the sign of the Creative.
    He toils in the sign of the Abysmal.
    He brings them to perfection in the sign of Keeping Still.

I Ching, *Book of Changes*

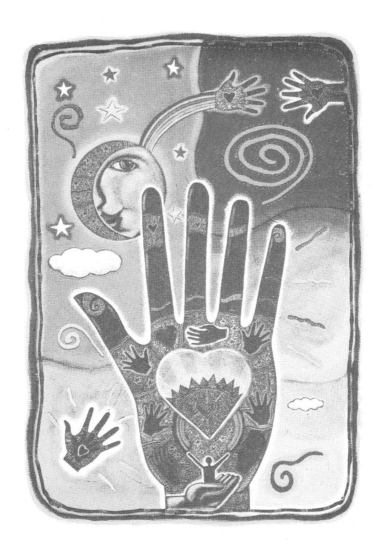

For you did form my inward parts,
      You knit me in my mother's womb.
I praise You for you are fearful and wonderful.
      Wonderful are your works!

You know me well;
      My frame is not hidden from you
When I was being made in secret
      Intricately wrought in the depth of the earth.

Your eye beheld my unformed substance.
      In Your Book is written, every one of them;
The days that are formed for me,
      Even those that have not yet passed.

How precious to me are Your thoughts, Oh God.
      How vast is the sum of them!
If I count them, they are more than the sand.
      When I awake I am still with You.

The Holy Bible, Psalm 139:13-18

The Serenity Prayer

God, grant me the Serenity
To Accept the things I cannot change,
    Courage to change the things I can,
And Wisdom to know the difference.

St. Francis of Assisi

Everything
the Power of the World
does is done in a circle. The sky is
round, and I have heard that the earth is
round like a ball, and so are all the stars. The
wind, in its greatest power whirls. Birds make
their own nests in a circle; theirs is the same religion as ours. The sun comes forth and goes down
again in a circle. The moon does the same, and both
are round. Even the seasons form a great wide circle in
their changing, and always come back again to where
they were. The life of a man is a circle from childhood
to childhood, and so it is in every thing where power
moves. Our tepees were round like the nests of birds,
and these were always set in a circle, the nation's
hoop, a nest of many nests, where the Great
Spirit meant for us to hatch our children.
ooo Black Elk, Sioux, from ooo
ooo *Black Elk Speaks* ooo

Mantras, psalms, hymns, and poems are a collect to God and symbolize the mandala. The mandala is an ancient spiritual symbol to the people of China and India. The psychologist who gave it new meaning in the occidental sense was Carl Gustav Jung. Jung was a Swiss contemporary of Freud and offers much information on the psyche and its relationship to mother, rebirth, and spirit.

Western civilization describes the mandala using Jung's expression, "the collective unconscious or the indwelling spiritual core of a person."

Western civilization describes the mandala using Jung's expression, "the collective unconscious or the indwelling spiritual core of a person." Every culture, no matter how primordial, gives expression to a spirit core of the human being in some way. In this work we use the mandala to represent the affirmation that is within us because we, as well as any human, have God and can tap the strength and the direction that the realization of God gives.

As mentioned previously, the "talking circle" of the Native American youngster is an example

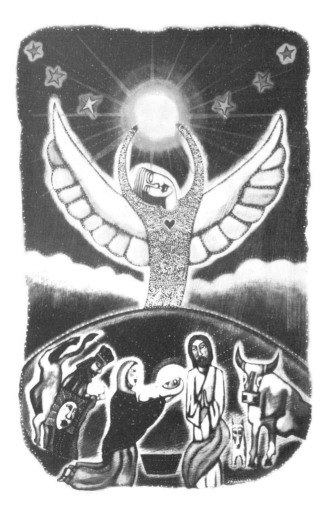

of communication with the wholeness of each person in their tribe. In the Christian tradition, Acts 17: 23 describes Saint Paul as he discovered a monument "To the Unknown God." Even though the Greeks had many gods, they were searching for a living relationship. The need for a relationship with God is universal. The unifying image of the mandala symbolizes the plea of our children for helpers who will listen to them. It is an appeal to realize the spiritual guidance of a living God of action as a part of daily life.

> **GOAL: To raise awareness of the mandala or sustaining spiritual core that nurtures the soul of a person and maintains emotional well-being.**

Objective One: Learn about the meaning of our given name, for it, like our heritage, is a positive affirmation of who we are.

Objective Two: Investigate the extremes within our personal mandala by graphic expression of our "worst fear" and our "best hope."

Objective Three: Examine the idea that "Life is fair;" or "Life is not fair."

Objective Four: Return to the genogram, the heritage circle, or the family tree and examine the expression of the mandala and our faith as our family passes it to us.

METHOD: Group process is the method of attaining cohesion of group members for peer support. Present the less threatening Modules One through Five to establish group trust. Use the "mandala" of Module Six to move from information and education to the personal and intimate stage of group work.

A theoretical "hierarchy of needs" was conceptualized by Abraham Maslow. Within the framework of a pyramid, Maslow shows that the broadest and most basic need fulfillment is biological in nature. This gratification includes areas of hunger, thirst, comfort and sex. The areas of safety, belongingness, esteem and self-actualization form the second through the fifth layers of the pyramid with self-actualization at the pinnacle. Self-actualization, as Maslow describes it, is what healthy young people determine they are capable of becoming; and, working toward that goal, they are willing to sacrifice immediate need fulfillment. Maslow also notes the adjustment problems that become ingrained when youth are not self-actualized. The desire for instant gratification leads to risk-taking behaviors. Barriers of poverty and poor adult role models put self-actualization out of reach so youngsters never realize a well-built hierarchal pyramid. In other words, even basic needs are not met and youth are robbed of a fulfilling life.

A recent article in *Public Health Reports* describes focus group research supported jointly by grants from the Public Health Service and the Departments of Education, Justice, and Transportation. The focus groups included youth who practiced high risk behaviors, but lacked an awareness of the motivation for these behaviors. One excerpt from this 1991 study states, "The youth said that knowing why (high risk) practices were harmful was not enough to help them change the behavior." The need for skill building and support systems to reinforce what they learned about changing their behaviors was very important.

Ranking of human needs via anecdotal data and questionnaires completed within the focus groups showed a hierarchy of needs similar to Maslow's description. The areas of belongingness and self-esteem were addressed. "Many participants said they wanted to talk to someone they could trust, who knew what they were going through." The group leaders found that a need for home and family support ranked first as a need that the youth identified.

Ranking second in importance as a category of need was that of spiritual provision. This can best be expressed by the following direct quotes from members of the focus groups:

"God is your number one priority. Without God, you won't be able to breathe. . . . "You wouldn't have none of the things on that list."

"You need to be close to God."

"If you don't have friends, God's your friend."

The idea of a spiritual core or mandala is difficult to express, yet these youth voiced a need with which many youth identify.

The concept of the mandala is easier to reach by feeling than by thinking. Pregnant or other high risk groups of teens approach the working stage of group with more negative than positive feelings about themselves. The goal of Module Six is to use a teen's indwelling spirit to raise positive hopes and dreams. At the outset of the working stage it is important to discuss fears, depression, lost expectations, and shattered dreams so they can be acknowledged, processed, and replaced with the realization of a strong positive spiritual core that supports life.

Using water colors, crayons, color pencils or markers, ask the students to draw two circles. Within the first circle they are to express their "worst fear" of life as a teenager. Within the second circle they are to express their "best hope" of what adolescence symbolizes personally. The personal nature of this material requires a long time to process. The group facilitator needs to arrange a longer group meeting time to give participants time to manage their feelings.

Other media and exercises initiate sharing the mandala. Clay modeling or paper cut-outs are used to show family relationships as are family sculpting and journal writing. Journal entries about emotions do not come easily to many teens. Using a few minutes at the beginning of a session and asking for written response to a specific situation can help one begin. With this sharing, teens realize the emotional benefits that come with releasing feelings as they are put down on paper.

Because of their cognitive level of development, adolescents often think of life in concrete terms. They see the material quality of life as attainable or not and judge life "fair" or "not fair" based on this materialistic model. They explore other facets of life qualities through the mandala. There is the opportunity to acknowledge positive attributes within the teen, his or her partner, and the extended families.

Objective four encourages a teen volunteer to share his genogram. He will show how different characteristics within the family of origin have influenced sexuality or pregnancy and feelings of belongingness. A chalk board, an overhead, or a piece of butcher paper and a marker work well for diagraming the genogram. The essence of the mandala can go with the members as they close each successive session with a group hug and the prayer, *"God grant me the Serenity to Accept the things I cannot change, Courage to Change the things I can, and Wisdom to Know the difference."*

QUESTIONS FOR CONSIDERATION:

1)   Is the quest to find one's spiritual core a primitive calling?

2)   Who is Black Elk and what is the import of his message?

3)   What is the significance of the statement of Black Elk, "The life of a man is a circle from childhood to childhood?"

4)   What movement endorsed the importance of the *Serenity Prayer* as a universal prayer? How does it affirm the significance of the mandala?

5)   Are there signs of cooperation among adults of the extreme conservative to the extreme liberal coming together for the welfare of adolescents and concerns of teen sexuality?

6)   Imagine, name, and discuss possible negative attitudes that might surface when a teen is expressing their "worst fear" about high risk behavior or the outcome of a teen pregnancy.

7)   Now imagine, name, and discuss positive attributes that may emerge when an adolescent is presenting his or her genogram.

8)   How does one handle a situation where a student is deeply moved or becomes intensely emotional about what is shared or what they feel is expected within the group?

9)   What's in a name? How do you feel about your name? Get a book about the meaning of names and discover the positive affirmations. Does it express how you feel about yourself ?

10) Reconsider your genogram. How does it reflect parts of your personal mandala that are passed down from generation to generation? What facets of your spirituality are affirmed?

MODULE SEVEN
ASSERTIVENESS

"Schroeder"

Schroeder recalled going through a tumultuous time when she got out of law school, went to work, and then started having babies. For a while she tried her hand at being a full-time mother and vividly remembered thinking one day, as she was feeding babies and watching Barbara Walters on TV, "Oh, my God. What have I done to my life? Will I ever be anything other than a peas pusher?"

The Schroeder spoken of in this scenario is the Pat Schroeder who went on to become the Congresswoman from Colorado and has served in the Congress of the United States for over two decades. In this excerpt from an interview for *Women In Power*, Pat Schroeder shows a side of herself that is appropriate to include in a book that speaks of women's - and men's - dilemmas with prevention, pregnancy, and parenting. We can hear any teen who is soon to be a parent say, "Oh, God, what have I done to my life?" and even, "Will I ever be anything other than a peas pusher?" Ms. Schroeder's matter-of-fact and unassuming attitude is an example of a person who is assertive. She is not submissive, nor is she aggressive. She considers her goals carefully and then garners support to attain her ambitions.

Becoming more assertive without being perceived as angry or negative is a new idea to adolescents. It is more important to teens to acquiesce and appear normal than to disagree and appear different from one's peers. Teens acquire assertiveness at different planes of awareness. For example, the teen who sees her friends smoke and feels the high when she joins them does not internalize the debits of the habit. However, that same teen may have experienced the death of a favorite aunt who died of lung cancer and may or may not view that consequence as a deterrent to her own activities.

People, including close family members who are key to teen growth sometimes voice the destructive "Ain't it a shame" language when talking to and about teens. Peers, parents, group leaders and any others who sincerely believe in what teens can do for themselves have unlocked a key to understanding teen development. Adults need to "just be there" as effective models of assertiveness without correcting teens or giving them advice.

> **GOAL: To define assertiveness as a positive behavioral trait that is essential to mature decision-making and to the developmental tasks of intimacy and independence.**

Objective One: Define assertiveness and discuss modeling, behavior rehearsal, and education that help a person become more honest and independent.

Objective Two: Discuss how adolescents learn appropriate intimacy and independence, the primary tasks of normal development for adolescents and young adults, as theorized by Erik Erikson.

Objective Three: Define self-efficacy and Albert Bandura's contributions to help teens be more assertive.

Objective Four: Study the contributions of Julian Rotter and his theory about a locus of control and individuals who are internally-directed or externally-directed.

Objective Five: Apply the Rathus Assertiveness Schedule to a practical study of assertiveness.

METHOD: One task of a program to prevent teen pregnancy is supporting the self-worth of teens to help them attain vocational, academic, and extracurricular success and to graduate from high school. The theories of psychosocial theorist Erik Erikson promote healthy psychosocial development. Erikson discussed eight life stages of development outlined on page 46. The task of adolescence is competency in identity versus role confusion. Erikson defines the task of identity as "connecting skills and interests to the formation of career objectives."

The task of the stage of young adulthood is characterized by the importance of intimacy versus isolation. Erikson further identifies the task of this stage as "committing oneself to another in an intimate relationship." Teens can use Erikson's information to confirm the value of assertiveness in pursuing the goals of identity and intimacy.

As illustrated by modeling, assertiveness gets its power from many different sources. We have already talked in Module Eight about the mandala as it expresses the strong spiritual core on which teens depend. A practical application of the mandala to assertiveness is the ability to love oneself. Self-love is often viewed by teens as indulgent and selfish. As an attribute, it is the basis for self-respect and a healthy desire to be assertive.

Albert Bandura, Julian Rotter, Spencer Rathus, and their current theories about assertiveness reflect the way different people view and use the trait of assertiveness. Bandura proposes that the degree of assertiveness depends on self-efficacy, a confidence in one's self that says, "If I think I can, I can. If I think I can't, I can't." About teen pregnancy he would say, "If I think I can avoid pregnancy as a teen, I can. If I think I cannot avoid teen pregnancy, I cannot."

Julian Rotter, a contemporary of Bandura, takes us one step further to a theory he expresses as "the internal locus of control or the external locus of control." Rotter asserts, "Some people are inner directed and learn from their mistakes without the direction of other people. Other people need the reflections of people's opinions to change behavior."

A teen who recognizes cause and effect and applies it to himself or herself internalizes a newly discovered thought or feeling; that teen has an "internal locus of control." The teen, such as the girl who knows about the correlation of smoking and lung cancer to the death of her favorite aunt may still choose to smoke. She views it as a "cool" activity to do with friends who model the smoking behavior. The mind set of others influences her and they externally motivate her. This teen operates from an "external locus of control."

> **A teen who recognizes cause and effect and applies it to himself or herself internalizes a newly discovered thought or feeling; that teen has an "internal locus of control."**

Spencer Rathus' study of assertiveness grew out of a curiosity about the assertiveness of women. Rathus contends that all periods of history show established boundaries for the behavior of women and how they assert themselves. Documented support for this idea dates back to the work of G.W. Allport in the United States in the early nineteen hundreds. It is still a new idea that women are learning to become assertive and that it is socially acceptable feminine behavior to be assertive.

Rathus saw the need to develop a tool specific to test assertiveness and gains made as the attribute is modeled, rehearsed and practiced. Rathus asked students in his psychology classes to "record behaviors the students would have liked to exhibit but refrained from exhibiting because of fear of aversive social consequences." These suggestions and other assertiveness items from student diaries were incorporated in the Rathus Assertiveness Schedule.

The Rathus Assertiveness Schedule (RAS) on page 47 is a quick test of assertiveness that has reliability and validity in English-speaking countries. One can administer it just after establishing a group. Pretesting a teen as group work begins is important because assertiveness changes with modeling, rehearsal, education, and practice. Post-testing with the RAS means administering it again before group closure to see if the student has become more or less assertive or has experienced a change in attitudes toward career goals and management of intimacy.

To administer the test, choose a quiet environment with no distractions. Before the test, review any words within the test that may cause confusion or may not be readily recognized by a student. Explain and make a display of the Likert scale of response. Read each statement clearly two times, giving time for response. Move on to the next statement until all statements have been read. Responses may be scored individually. If the schedule is used with large groups of teens, the Likert response scale can be adapted to computer data cards, marked with a number two pencil, and scored automatically. Note that the asterisks behind selected statements indicate a reversed item. The process is repeated for post-testing.

If reading levels are established, one can use adapted versions of the schedule; the Simple Rathus Assertiveness Schedule has been created to reliably assess subjects with a low reading age. The Modified Rathus Assertiveness Schedule has been created to allow testing of students as young as eleven years of age.

Erik Erikson's Stages of Development

Time Period	Life Point	Developmental Task
Infancy (0-1)	Trust versus Mistrust	Trusting mother and environment
Early Childhood (2-3)	Autonomy versus Shame and Doubt	Desire to make choices and follow through on choices
Preschool Years (4-5)	Initiative versus Guilt	Adding planning to choices; becoming active
Grammar School Years (6-12)	Industry versus Inferiority	Becoming absorbed in tasks and productive pursuits
Adolescence	Identity versus Role Confusion	Connecting skills and interests to formation of career objectives
Young Adulthood	Intimacy versus Isolation	Committing oneself to another in an intimate relationship
Middle Adulthood	Generativity versus Stagnation	Needing to be needed; guiding younger generation; striving to be creative
Late Adulthood	Integrity versus Despair	Accepting one's place in the life cycle; achieving wisdom and dignity

Rathus Assertiveness Schedule

Directions: Indicate how characteristic or descriptive each of the following statements is of you by using the code given below:

+3 very characteristic of me, extremely descriptive
+2 rather characteristic of me, quite descriptive
+1 somewhat characteristic of me, slightly descriptive
-1 somewhat uncharacteristic of me, slightly nondescriptive
-2 rather uncharacteristic of me, quite nondescriptive
-3 very uncharacteristic of me, extremely nondescriptive

____01. Most people seem to be more aggressive and assertive than I am.*
____02. I have hesitated to make or accept dates because of "shyness."*
____03. When the food served at a restaurant is not done to my satisfaction, I complain to the waiter or waitress.
____04. I am careful to avoid hurting other people's feelings, even when I feel that I have been injured.*
____05. If a salesman has gone to considerable trouble to show me merchandise which is not quite suitable, I have a difficult time in saying "No."*
____06. When I am asked to do something, I insist upon knowing why.
____07. There are times when I look for a good, vigorous argument.
____08. I strive to get ahead as well as most people in my position.
____09. To be honest, people often take advantage of me.*
____10. I enjoy starting a conversation with new acquaintances and strangers.
____11. I often don't know what to say to attractive persons of the opposite sex.*
____12. I will hesitate to make phone calls to business establishments and institutions.*
____13. I would rather apply for a job or for admission to a college by writing letters than by going through with personal interviews.*
____14. I find it embarrassing to return merchandise.*
____15. If a close and respected relative were annoying me, I would smother my feelings rather than express annoyance.*
____16. I have avoided asking questions for fear of sounding stupid.*
____17. During an argument I am sometimes afraid that I will get so upset that I will shake all over.*
____18. If a famed and respected lecturer makes a statement which I think is incorrect, I will have the audience hear my point of view as well.
____19. I avoid arguing over prices with clerks and salesmen.*
____20. When I have done something important or worthwhile, I manage to let others know about it.
____21. I am open and frank about my feelings.
____22. If someone has been spreading false and bad stories about me, I see him (her) as soon as possible to "have a talk" about it.
____23. I often have a hard time saying "No."*
____24. I tend to bottle up emotions rather than make a scene.*
____25. I complain about poor service in a restaurant or elsewhere.
____26. When I am given a compliment, I sometimes just don't know what to say.*
____27. If a couple near me in a theatre or at a lecture were conversing rather loudly, I would ask them to be quiet.
____28. Anyone attempting to push ahead of me in a line is in for a good battle.
____29. I am quick to express an opinion.
____30. There are times when I just can't say anything.*

Total score obtained by adding numerical responses to each item, after changing signs of reversed items.
*Reversed item.

QUESTIONS FOR CONSIDERATION:

1)   Study Erikson's theory of human development and apply it to three people who are at different levels or stages of development. What uniqueness do you see at each stage?

2)   Now take three persons within the same stage of development; are they about the same or drastically different in their viewpoints and life pursuits?

3)   Compare and contrast the ideas of Rathus, Rotter, and Bandura as they relate to self-efficacy and assertiveness.

4)   Is the Rathus Assertiveness Schedule an effective tool to measure assertiveness in terms of validity, reliability, and norm referencing?

5)   Are peers more important to an adolescent than are family members?

6)   In your view, are teen males more or less assertive than teen females, what are the reasons for your answer?

7)   Might a person who functions from an external locus of control become a person who functions from an internal locus of control?

8)   "Self-efficacy can be a life or death matter as it applies to teen sexuality." Why is this statement a reality in today's society?

9)   There is a realization among women that modern day behavioral theorists are of the male gender. What bearing does this have on outcomes of teen development and answers to teen sexuality?

10) Choose a female author of behavioral ideas such as Michele Weiner-Davis who wrote *Divorce-Busting*, or Mary Pipher who wrote *Reviving Ophelia*, or Harriet Goldhor-Lerner who wrote *The Dance of Anger*, and rewrite Erik Erikson's Stages of Development from a female point of view.

MODULE EIGHT
ALCOHOL, TOBACCO, DRUG USE AND ABUSE

"Quality of Life"

The cell phone chirped like an annoying canary. Ms. Deenan eased the phone out of her belt loop and answered it as she hurried down the hall. A man's voice asked courteously for the nurse. "I'll transfer to my office phone if you'll wait a minute," Ms. Deenan replied as the bell rang and students flooded the hallway pushing, pestering and jostling each other in lively nonsense as they moved from class to class.

"Yes," responded Ms. Deenan, to the concerned parent on the other end of the line. "I did talk to Alex about his chewing tobacco last Friday." A silent pause hung in the air uncertainly, then Alex's father asked, "What right does a school nurse have to bring up chewing, anyway? Alex was very upset when he came home. He talked to my wife and me right away. He is not hiding *anything* from us."

Another long pause and Ms. Deenan, feeling queasy inside, responded. "I can answer your concern with a story; it happened only three months ago. I was talking to a parent; a conversation with her daughter led to questions about the girl's use of alcohol. As in your situation, the mother believed it was not my concern to be talking to her daughter."

"Not even one month later that same girl and her boyfriend were returning from 'a cabin party' on a Sunday morning. The kegger, which had started on a balmy autumn evening the night before, was ending as the two young people headed to town and their Sunday jobs that did not start until the afternoon shift. Lightheaded and sleepy, the girl was driving down the highway. In a split second her life became a nightmare as she swerved into the path of an oncoming car. The lone driver was killed instantly. Neither of the young people died - they were perfectly unharmed with blood alcohol levels of .125."

"If I talked to your young person, take it seriously. I only want to be of some help to him, I do not do it maliciously or without good cause. We are concerned about all substance abuse. It **is** a personal call and a first step. There are other avenues and other people to help your son if you feel he needs it; I would be happy to help you with those resources."

Drug and alcohol use and abuse rob many teens of their futures and sometimes their lives. It is worth noting, by their own reports, that young men and women lose inhibitions when they are using and abusing alcohol, tobacco, and other drugs. It is often the time that young women become pregnant. If they were not under the influence of alcohol, they would choose to abstain from risky sexual encounters.

GOAL: To increase teen awareness that any alcohol, tobacco, or drug use, whether legal or illicit, is physically abusive to the body.

Objective One: Discuss the high risk behavior of alcohol, tobacco, and other drug (ATOD) use and abuse and how it applies to teen sexuality.

Objective Two: Look at the genogram and trace specific instances of family patterns of use and abuse and the outcomes.

Objective Three: Instill the idea in both pregnant parents that their use of alcohol, tobacco and other drugs can be temporarily or permanently damaging to their baby.

Objective Four: Define and discuss the placental barrier and show how the characteristics of chemicals called teratogens are harmful to mother and fetus.

METHOD: Two developmental attitudes that make teens more vulnerable to unintended pregnancy are invincibility and immaturity. Youths do not live life avoiding high risk behaviors. Risk-taking behaviors increase with drinking, decreasing inhibitions and use of birth control, and increasing the likelihood of pregnancy.

Societal norms are strong regarding drinking and pregnancy. The norm motivates teen women to stop using to protect the unborn child. Early detection of pregnancy allows early education and support to protect the mother and the fetus. The risks of birth defects are highest between the fifth and tenth week of fetal life. Helpful "no use" messages to teens include the statement: "If you are sexually active and have missed a period, do not continue to smoke or drink."

> **"If you are sexually active and have missed a period, do not continue to smoke or drink."**

Information about chemical use and abuse to teenagers is age-related. Gateway drugs such as cigarettes, marijuana, and beer are the illicit drugs most frequently abused by teens. Adolescent behavior is not usually restrained. Drinking to get drunk or toking to get stoned is the result of adolescent chemical use whether teens are experimenting, socially using, or addicted. Other age-related legal drugs commonly used by adolescents are Acutane and doxycycline for acne. Caffeinated beverages and antidepressant medications such as Zoloft, Prozac, and amitriptyline are used for depression. Ritalin and Dexedrine are used for attention-deficit and hyperactivity disorders. The benefits of these legal prescriptions may outweigh their disadvantages; however, their side effects do not promote healthy cell growth.

The genogram of an individual can show the vulnerability of a teen to family addictions; the importance of a drug free environment extends to friends and family whose support is vital if a chemically dependent teen is to stop using and abusing alcohol, tobacco, and other drugs.

Risk Factors in Fetal Development

Cultural, societal, and personal factors influence how a woman views her health, her womanhood, and her pregnancy. Surveys by questionnaire have shown that drinking and drug use decreases a person's inhibitions. Diminished inhibitions decrease the likelihood of using birth control and increase the likelihood of conception. However, there is a strong societal message that a pregnant person should stop using any alcohol, tobacco, or other drugs if she is pregnant.

The risks of birth defects are highest between the fifth and the tenth week of pregnancy. Most teens do not know or they deny that they are pregnant during the peak time of fetal risk for birth defects. The message that can reduce those risks is: "If you have missed a period, do not drink, smoke, or use legal or illegal drugs of any kind." The elements or substances that interrupt normal gestation or alter genetic matter to produce a birth defect are called teratogens. The following teratogens, used legally or illegally by adolescents, increase the risk of a birth defect.

1. Doxycycline and other antibiotics - Are used for teen-age acne and chlamydia infections; doxycycline can cause skeletal and dental weaknesses or defects in a fetus.

2. Acutane - A prescription drug used to treat acne; causes problems to skeletal development of a fetus.

3. Cocaine, Ritalin, Dexedrine, Antidepressants - These substances are stimulants and in varying quantity can cause abruptio placenta, preterm labor, racing fetal heartbeat.

4. Opiates - Morphine, codeine, demerol, and heroin are substances that physically and emotionally kill pain. These substances slow fetal heartbeat and can cause stillbirths and low birth weight babies.

5. Nicotine, Tobacco, Marijuana - These substances constrict vessels to decrease blood supply to the fetus. When a pregnant female uses tobacco products, poisons cross the placental barrier and reach the fetus. One such substance is carbon monoxide that acts by replacing maternal blood oxygen. Oxygen starvation results and proper metabolism of nutrients does not take place. The baby is undernourished and fails to thrive to potential.

6. Alcohol - Alcohol is found in beer, wine, hard liquor, and some elixir-based medications for treating asthma. This substance crosses the placental barrier and bathes the fetal brain and body cells in a toxic environment that either kills or reduces the ability of fetal cells to perform normally. In addition, the energy provided by alcohol is not nutritious so starvation or the lack of food for proper growth results. Alcohol consumption during pregnancy is known to promote fetal alcohol effects (FAE) and/or fetal alcohol syndrome (FAS).

QUESTIONS FOR CONSIDERATION:

1)   Is there such a thing as "responsible" alcohol, tobacco, and drug use? Is there such a thing as an "alcoholic" or "drug-addicted" adolescent?

2)   Does alcohol, tobacco, and drug use change the physical growth of an adolescent body? Does the use of ATOD affect the emotional growth and maturity of adolescents?

3)   Do alcohol, tobacco, and other drugs affect an adolescent body in the same way as they change an adult body?

4)   Studies show a rise in teen use of tobacco products. See "Current Statistics" on page 114. What responsibility rests with tobacco companies who use sex appeal to attract teens to smoking and chewing tobacco?

5)   Do the investigation and reporting of teen alcohol, tobacco, and drug abuse contradict laws about confidentiality? Is the discussion of alcohol abuse with a teen an invasion of their privacy and a violation of recently enacted human rights protection?

6)   In your view, is a teen "alcoholic" or "drug addict" a sick person in need of health care, an impaired individual in need of remediation and rehabilitation, or a potential criminal in need of incarceration? What if his or her use of alcohol or other drugs leads to other crimes?

7)   Is the increased legalized use of Ritalin and other prescribed drugs for attention deficit disorder a drug problem in our schools?

8)   Interview an obstetrical doctor to see how he or she manages the nausea, headaches, and urinary tract infections of a pregnant teen. Name the medications that they prescribe and discuss their side effects.

9)   Societal pressures about responsibility to the fetus compel a teen mother to be drug free during pregnancy; are teen fathers drug free? Identify the important messages fathers convey when they remain drug free; discuss differences of behavior in drug use versus nonuse.

10) Become aware of and collect periodical and newspaper articles that report damage to sperm and semen from alcohol, tobacco, and drug abuse.

MODULE NINE
SELF-WORTH AND CODEPENDENCY

"The Reality of A National Statistic"

The rate of births to teens in the United States has averaged about 13 percent annually for the past five years. Statistics present teen mothers or fathers who are more apt to be poor than rich, have a 50% chance of seeking and receiving adequate prenatal care, have a 35% to 60% chance of having a repeat pregnancy in the teen years, have a 20% chance of delivering a preterm or a low birth weight baby, who are receiving partial help from the family 75% of the time, and are 100% likely to drop out of high school if their dilemma is not recognized, acknowledged, and remedied.

To make this information more indelible, there is Kate and her boyfriend Sean. I met Kate in her first year of high school. Kate's pale profile was like a silhouette against her thick, dark hair. She had fulfilled the mother-role in her family for a long time. Her biological mother, Anna, was singly raising four children on a secretary's salary. Anna had divorced Kate's father because "he was drinking too much," a minimalization of the father's outrageous alcoholism that led to the mosaic of family risks we are discussing.

Kate's family expected Kate to have adult insight into her siblings' physical and emotional needs and to take care of them. Anna was taking care of her pain through Alanon. She frequently accused Kate of being "just like her Dad." Kate had an alcohol possession fine for being picked up at a kegger with her friends. This was not Kate's first incident of underage drinking and others occurred repeatedly throughout Kate's sophomore year of high school.

Kate sought help outside her family and her worst fear was confirmed; she was pregnant. Kate had been dating her current boyfriend, Sean, for three months. He was employed at a local fast food restaurant. Kate's immediate family history of alcoholism and poor access to medical care put her baby at risk for the delivery of a preterm or low birth weight baby. Nevertheless, Kate never missed school and her grades were of honor roll quality. In the middle of her pregnancy she decided to take advantage of a support group. Kate became aware of potential for change in herself and in her relationships. She attended the group faithfully and during the following six months began prenatal care with a local physician on a reduced fee basis.

Kate gave birth to a seven-pound baby girl in the middle of her junior year. She maintained her school attendance. She graduated, although she did drop from honor roll status. Without the support of her peers Kate knows she would not have made it through a troublesome time in her life. She came to terms with her mother over the accusations that Anna had hurled at Kate over the years. There was much work to do, but both mother and daughter had community support to carry them over the rough spots.

GOAL: To nurture self-reliance and healthy interdependence.

Objective One: Define, compare, and contrast interdependence and codependency.

Objective Two: Increase knowledge of the visible and hidden self using the Jo-Hari Window.

Objective Three: Review assertiveness, inner direction, and spiritual values.

Objective Four: Explore the need of grandparent involvement in teen pregnancy.

Objective Five: Understand the mental health benefits of using a self-care contract with a friend or counselor.

METHOD: The reasons why adolescents find themselves in an unplanned pregnancy vary. In some families, teen pregnancy is a family standard because values and expectations have not changed from one generation to the next. In other situations, the possibility of "accidental" pregnancies is increased given our present social standards and the increased amount of time adolescents spend with their peers. In yet other families, drug or alcohol-induced invincibility, as an underlying condition of some pregnancies, arises from dysfunctional family patterns that foster codependency. In those families, teen pregnancy is a symptom of unresolved family problems.

Return to the genogram of Module Three as we discuss codependency and the chief enabler. Codependent persons can be thought of as those who lose their selfhood because they sustain their identity only through the life and personality of another family member or members. Interdependent persons, on the other hand, are those who nurture each other through success and tragedy but do not lose their own personality or life identity in that process. "Get a life!" is the teen expression that acknowledges codependency and its remedy.

Family roadblocks to discussing and accepting a teen's sexuality are often grounded in codependency. Codependency stunts the growth of intimacy and independence, and the young people from such a family framework have not had the luxury of devoting time to thinking about their own welfare. As children and young adolescents, they are caught in the role of care-taking or parenting their parents and their siblings. The search for intimacy and a way to "get out" of an undesirable family puts them in relationships that they were never taught to manage. Protection is not a word in their vocabulary because no one ever protected them or modeled the protection of abstinence or birth control. The myth that having a baby fills a loveless void thrives in this situation.

Often questions about feelings, expectations within the family, and education about intimacy, abstinence, and birth control to prevent pregnancy and second pregnancies are easier if approached in an individual setting. As trust levels increase, the person can be privately encouraged to share his or her situation in the group setting. Group discussions can challenge unhealthy choices and support healthy ones. A group that fosters positive attitudes and acceptance shows that they can love a person even if his choices are not acceptable. The Rathus

Assertiveness Schedule repeated after group work has been progressing shows increased assertiveness and self-worth. Discussing these positive gains with group members is a good way to review the importance of voicing feelings, coming to terms with differences within the group, and accepting one's imperfections and life's unfairness.

The Jo-Hari Window on page 56 is a simple chart to aid in the discussions of self-disclosure. It has two columns, "known to me" and "unknown to me;" and two rows, "known to others" and "unknown to others;" thus there are four distinct areas of the window. The Jo-Hari Window can be used in individual counseling as a teaching tool. In group work it is effective because members describe themselves with appropriate guidance from the Window in the categories of: 1) what I know about myself that others also know about me, 2) what I know about me that others do not know about me, 3) what I do not know about myself but others know about me, and 4) what is unknown both to myself and to others. The simple outline of the Jo-Hari Window can be copied on poster board and used by the group as a discussion tool.

Self-disclosure is based on trust. Teens practice it in the spirit of self-improvement and self-empowerment. The soul-searching that teens do among themselves as "Why did this happen to me?" is answered when teens share issues of emotional stress and discover spiritual answers. Caring about each other can be modeled and practiced through use of the Self-Care Contract on page 57. Group members pair and study the contract. They share feelings with each other in or out of group meetings. After sharing and discussing the contract, each partner signs and dates it. Members also have each other's phone numbers when support is needed outside of group meeting time.

Jo-Hari Window

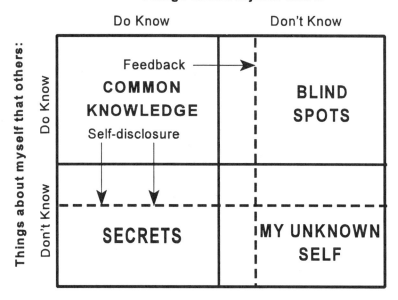

Common Knowledge - Things about myself that I know and others know about me as well. Information and feelings here are safe such as "My friends and I like to drive my blue Datsun to school." Discussion about changes in this area are not threatening.

Secrets - Things I know about myself but others do not know about me. For instance, an embarrassing detail would be, "My family can not afford to buy braces for my teeth." A secret such as one about sexual abuse may be much more threatening. These areas may or may not be open to discussion depending on trust level changes within a group.

Blind Spots - Things about myself I do not know but others do know about me. Others may see you as tired or unresponsive. However, you do not feel this way inside, and you do not know that others see you this way. When trust levels are high and people love each other despite discouraging characteristics, they share these observations to promote self-improvement.

Unknown Self - Things about myself I do not know and that others do not know about me. Areas that are repressed because they may contain disturbing revelations or demand the use of one's self-actualizing talents.

Self-Care Contract

1.   I will nurture and protect myself. I will not provoke anyone else to hurt me.

2.   I will respect myself and others and act in a responsible way. I will not harm any other person.

3.   I will not run away physically or emotionally.   I will stay, work through my feelings, thoughts, and behaviors.   I will own and solve my problems.

4.   I will not get sick or go crazy.   Instead, I will be and become sane and healthy and work through problems responsibly.

5.   I will not be passive or let things happen "to me."   I will react to my own and others' thoughts, feelings, and behaviors.

6.   I will take responsibility for my actions, but not for the actions of others.

Name_____   Date_____

Witness_____   Date_____

Directions For Use

1.   Pair up. Repeat each point above to your partner. Your partner will listen to you until he/she believes what you are saying. It may take several times and the more your repeat it, the more you feel the truth in what you are saying.

2.   This contract is a real way to begin self-care. Practice it in your group and self-care will become a part of your life.

QUESTIONS FOR CONSIDERATION:

1)   Are self-worth and codependency inversely correlated?

2)   Is it politically correct to encourage use of the *Serenity Prayer* for group closure?

3)   Controversy exists about offering support groups in school. What are the concerns? Identify advantages and disadvantages of this offering and discuss your examples.

4)   Read the introduction to *The Transparent Self* by Sidney M. Jourard and comment on what his work did for the progress of support groups.

5)   "Disclosure helps people discover their spiritual strength and their ability to use it." How does *The Serenity Prayer* affirm the preceding statement?

6)   Why is the statement "I will not provoke anyone else to hurt me," included in the self-care contract?

7)   What type of response in a passive-aggressive teen may be apparent to others in the "blind spot," but could be a behavior a teen does not recognize within herself or himself?

8)   Is it a myth that a baby fills a loveless void for a parenting teen?

9)   Discuss the pros and cons of "welfare" programs for the pregnant and parenting teen as to codependency.

10) Do self-contained child care programs offered through school or federal funding foster interdependency? Why? Why not?

MODULE TEN
BIRTH CONTROL AND SEXUALLY TRANSMITTED DISEASES

"Turning Crisis Into Remedy"

Teens seeking help about birth control are afraid. Fear that an untimely pregnancy has already occurred is at the root of the distress. Nevertheless, all is not lost because of this situation. First, it is fact that periods quit coming more often as a response to stress than to pregnancy. The health questionnaire is used to track the outcomes of pregnancy testing. It shows that about two-thirds of the teen women who refer themselves to help outside the family are not menstruating because the stress of imagined pregnancy is great enough to stop periods. Inversely, however, that means that about a third of teens are pregnant when they think they are.

...it is a fact that periods quit coming more often as a response to stress than to pregnancy.

Second, the disclosed fact of being sexually active can work in the young person's favor. Hidden behavior becomes open and available for remedy. Also, as described previously, the youngsters need to begin open discussion with their family of support. Promoting openness in family communication is stressed in the health questionnaire.

Thirdly, birth control is often not birth control at all. Concern about pregnancy gives an opportunity to share the need for protection against HIV/AIDS and other sexually transmitted diseases. Education about the symptoms and testing for sexually transmitted diseases is available to anyone who is sexually active, but it is most important to anyone who does not know their partner's sexual history.

Finally, if you are dealing with a teen who is pregnant, remember some areas of the United States have a repeat pregnancy rate of 35% to 60% in the teen years. If your program exists solely for reducing repeat pregnancy in the teen years, you have made a great contribution to reducing or preventing untimely repetitions.

> **GOAL: To create a teen environment that invites the discussion of birth control and sexually transmitted disease.**

Objective One: Explore "normal" feelings about intimacy, jealousy, control, boundaries, and motivation in teen relationships.

Objective Two: Discuss life choices and the option of abstinence for birth control and protection against sexually transmitted disease.

Objective Three: Learn about methods of birth control, their effectiveness, and their side effects.

Objective Four: Learn common terms used to discuss venereal disease.

Objective Five: Identify bacterial and viral infections of the reproductive system and define their characteristics.

Objective Six: Understand the importance of preventing sexually transmitted disease.

METHOD: Depending on the makeup of your teen group, you will have discussed intimacy, jealousy, control, boundaries, and motivation in previous modules. A review of these modules as they apply to birth control and sexually transmitted disease might be helpful.

Sharing a current, well-written brochure helps accurately address birth control concerns. Identifying and naming parts of the reproductive system are part of the discussion of birth control. Group work and the development of trust allows discussion and affirms caring enough about oneself to be responsible about protection. Handouts for discussing birth control are found on pages 63 to 67. For further resources use the "Resource Guide" on page 115.

> **Because teens have the choice of healthy abstinence, making it part of the discussion of birth control is important.**

Because teens have the choice of healthy abstinence, making it part of the discussion of birth control is important. The reason abstinence is qualified as "honest" or not on the chart on birth control, page 66, is that there is a point of conjecture as one explores the nature of teen sexuality and the teen's view of abstinence. In the article "Will Kids Buy Abstinence?" from the *Virginia Journal of Education*, Jerald Newberry, who oversees a family life curriculum in Fairfax County, Virginia says, "If kids are going to buy into abstinence, and if it's going to be a meaningful buy-in, they have to have enough information to say, 'I don't want to put myself at risk. I can have meaningful relationships without giving this piece of me away.'" Further, Newberry states, "We don't just say, 'Don't have sex because I say not to.' We'll say, 'Don't do this, and now let's do an activity to talk about why.'"

Newberry's ideas are affirmed by Carolyn Elliott, a former biology teacher who also defines, teaches about, and affirms abstinence within her biology curriculum. Elliott states, "If you look into the eyes of these kids, get into intelligent conversations with them, and give them correct information, you can make a case for abstinence and a lot more of them will choose it."

Newberry and Elliott have discussed abstinence in the sense of good physical and mental health and the fact that abstaining from sexual intercourse is normal behavior in the teen years. However, if a teen is already sexually active and dealing with venereal disease, supposed pregnancy, or diagnosed pregnancy, abstinence has an entirely different meaning. Teens in those situations may practice abstinence for unhealthy reasons such as self-punishment, fear, and guilt. Abstinence can begin anytime, leading to the idea of *secondary virginity* or the permission to forgive oneself for past actions and start over.

In situations where teen sexuality includes untimely pregnancy, venereal disease, or abortion, the discussion of birth control still includes abstinence. Encourage a discussion comparing feelings before intercourse with feelings after intercourse or a teen pregnancy. Examples of concerns that arise when honest feelings are expressed include the following: 1) body image and a jealousy that the fellow remains attractive and unattached while the young woman carries the baby, the venereal disease, or the trauma of abortion, 2) boundary issues and limits that exist because a couple have a baby together without the benefit of marriage, 3) control and financial concern that would not be part of a teen's life if there were not a pregnancy or ongoing treatment for a sexually transmitted disease, and 4) motivation to use birth control from a perspective that did not exist before sexual activity and pregnancy.

Private doctors' offices, Family Planning, and Planned Parenthood are agencies that will provide a guest speaker on birth control measures, including abstinence and counseling. Different states have programs that address abstinence. Concrete questions about availability, side effects, and extent of pregnancy protection are also concerns commonly addressed by the speaker.

A 1996 press release from the Center for Disease Control in Atlanta, Georgia, reported the work of Dr. Robert Pinner. Dr. Pinner conducted a study of every death certificate filed from 1980 to 1992. The mortality rate from infections rose from forty-one deaths per 100,000 people in 1980 to sixty-five per 100,000 in 1995. The AIDS virus accounted for most of the jump. Put another way, "when Pinner included HIV-related deaths, infectious disease mortality rose 22 percent."

In the same release, Nobel laureate Joshua Lederberg, said, "Infectious diseases are on a global rebound and the world is more vulnerable than ever before. The development of antibiotics once had doctors predicting infectious diseases would be conquered by now. Instead, in the past decade new infections such as the AIDS virus suddenly began killing hundreds of thousands; older diseases like tuberculosis returned and bacteria began evolving to defy treatment."

In the same breath, Lederberg emphasized, "This does not mean people should panic. The findings should persuade world governments and drug makers to fund research and fight back, and doctors to stop over-prescribing antibiotics, a practice that boosts drug-resistant bacteria."

The preceding discussion clarifies a rising concern of teen sexuality that dwarfs the concern of teen pregnancy. To prevent or reduce venereal disease, additional counsel from doctors and other health care professionals, community leaders, and parents can focus on abstinence messages. It is "normal" behavior to be abstinent from sexual intercourse in the teen years. Another message to sexually active teens includes supporting monogamous relationships where both persons have been tested for HIV/AIDS and other sexually transmitted diseases. Responsible sex education includes thorough discussion and encouragement of birth control methods that concurrently reduce the risk of sexually transmitted disease. Parents and mentoring adults who have not abdicated their place as role models can provide this education.

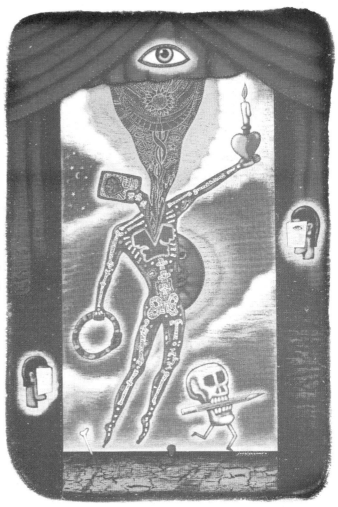

A Quick Index of Sexually Transmitted Diseases

STD	WHAT SIGNS TO WATCH FOR	HOW DO YOU GET THIS DISEASE?	WHAT HAPPENS WITHOUT TREATMENT/TYPE OF EFFECTIVE TREAT- MENT?
Chlamydia (Has viral and bacterial qualities.) Also called NGU or nongonococcal urethritis.	Signs show 7-21 days after sex. Most women and some men have no symptoms. WOMEN: Discharge from vagina. Bleeding from vagina between periods. Burning or pain with passing urine. Pain in low abdomen, sometimes with fever and nausea. MEN: Watery, white or yellow drip from penis. Burning or pain when urinating.	Spread during vaginal, anal, and oral sex with someone who has chlamydia or NGU.	You can give chlamydia to your sexual partner. Chlamydia can lead to more serious STD. Reproductive organs can be damaged. Men and women can become sterile. A mother can pass chlamydia to her baby during childbirth. Treatable with antibiotics, test for resistance.
Genital Warts (viral)	Symptoms show 1-8 months after sex. Tiny bumpy warts on sex organs, anus. Warts enlarge and will not go away. Itching and burning around sex organs. If warts go away for a time, they stay in the body and come back.	Spread during intercourse with someone who has warts or the wart virus.	Warts are passed to sexual partner. More warts grow on top of each other . A mother with warts can give them to her baby during childbirth. Warts are precancerous growths. Warts cannot be cured.
Gonorrhea (bacterial)	Symptoms show 2-21 days after sex. Most women and some men have no symptoms. MEN: Thick yellow discharge from penis. WOMEN: Thick yellow discharge from vagina. Burning on urination and bowel movement. Abnormal bleeding or periods. Cramps, pain in low abdomen.	All intercourse with someone who has gonorrhea bacteria. Carrier may not show signs of disease.	You can pass gonorrhea to your sexual partner. Gonorrhaea is a gateway infection. Reproductive organs can be damaged and result in sterilty. Can cause heart trouble, skin disease, arthritis, and blindness. Treatable with antibiotics, test for resistance.
Hepatitis B (viral)	Symptoms show 1-9 months after contact with virus. May have no signs or mild signs only. Flu-like symptoms that don't go away. Extreme fatigue. Jaundice (yellow skin and mucous membranes). Dark urine, light-colored bowel movements.	Intercourse contact with carrier. Contact with infected blood and stool. Infected needle contact.	Can pass to sexual and needle partners. Some people recover completely. Can cause permanent liver damage. Can be transferred to baby during childbirth. Vaccinate for immunity. No cure for some.
Herpes (viral)	Signs show 1-30 days after intercourse. No symptoms or flu-like symptoms. Small, painful blisters on sex organs that last 1-3 weeks. Blisters come and go because virus is harbored in nerve tracts of infected person.	All intercourse contact with infected or viral carrier of herpes.	Can give herpes to sexual partner. Herpes cannot be cured. A mother can give herpes to baby during childbirth.
HIV/AIDS (viral)	Symptoms show several months to years after contact with the virus. Can be present for many years with no symptoms. Unexplained weight loss or tiredness. Flu-like feelings that do not go away. Diarrhea. White spots in the mouth. Yeast infections that won't go away. Secondary infections.	Spread during anal, oral. or vaginal intercourse with partner with HIV/AIDS. Contact with infected blood. Spread by needle partners.	Passed to sexual and needle partners. HIV/AIDS have no cure; most people die. HIV/AIDS crosses tissue barriers and thrives in the womb, during birth , and during breast-feeding to infect the fetus or baby.
Syphilis (bacterial)	1st Stage: Shows 3-12 weeks after sex. Painless red, rough sore on mouth, sex organs, breast, or fingers for 1-5 weeks. 2nd Stage: Symptoms show 1 week to 6 months after sore heals. Body rash. Flu-like feeling. Rash and flu continue. Permanent 3rd and 4th stages in all organs.	Spread by sexual contact with person with syphilis.	Can be passed to sexual partner. Syphilis is passed during childbirth or causes miscarriage. Can cause heart disease, brain damage, blindness or death in adults, children and babies.

Sex and the Single Teen

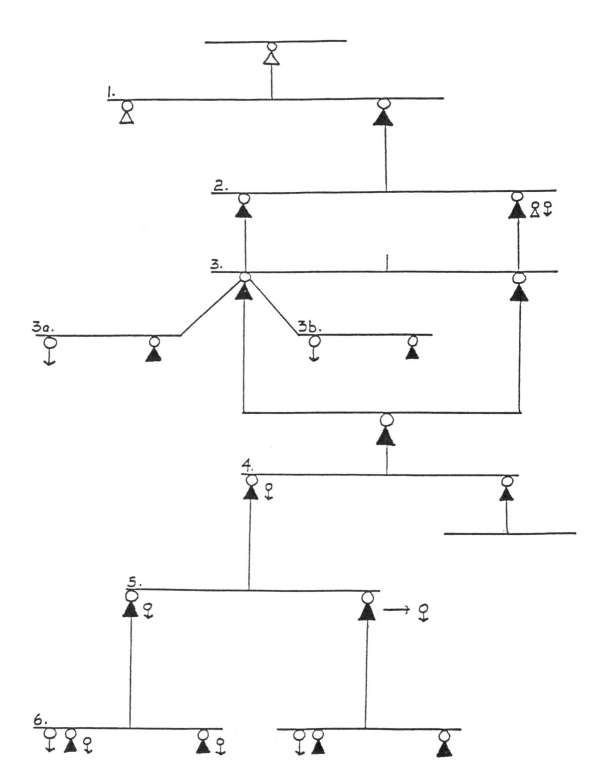

Sex and the Single Teen

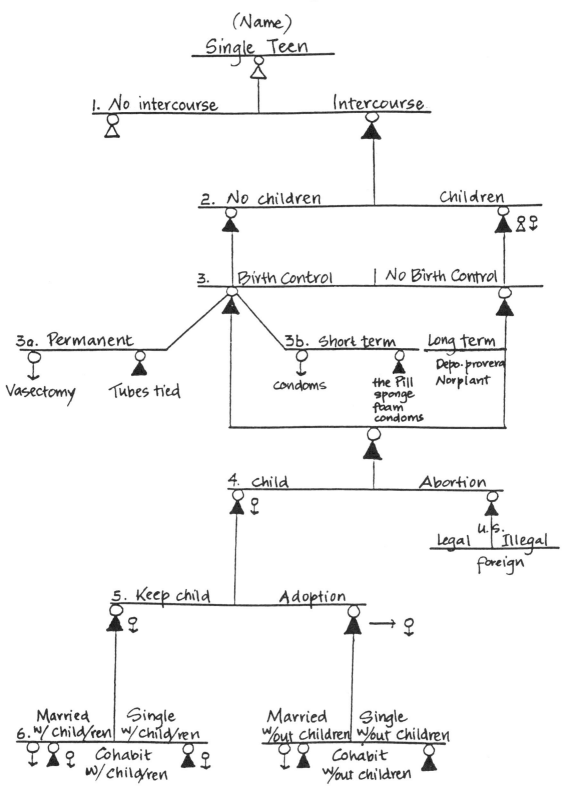

Birth Control Methods and Effectiveness

METHOD	EFFECTIVENESS/COST ideal-actual -teens		ADVANTAGES	DISADVANTAGES	PHYSICAL SIDE EFFECTS
Honest Abstinence	100%	0	No worry about pregnancy	Frustration? Self control	0%
Condoms	98%, 88%, 78 %	Low	No physical side effects	Interferes with spontaneity, planned	0%
The Pill	97%, 97%, ?	Med	Easy with good memory	Subject to abuse as used by teens	Nausea, weight gain, clots, breast cancer
Depo-Provera	99%, 99%, 99%	High	Easy, no planning needed	All physical side effects not known	Fetal complications, bone marrow depletion
Norplant	99%, 99%, 99%	High	Easy, no planning needed	Irreversible for five years, legal issues pending	Clotting, bone marrow depletion, breast cancer
Spermicidal Foam, Jelly, Sponges	90%, 80%, 70%	Low	Easy, few side effects	Effectiveness expires, plan to have available	Cervical irritation, precancerous lesions
IUD - Intra-uterine device	95% not used by teens	Med	Small worry about pregnancy	Some reports of painful menstruation	Negligible
Withdrawal	96%, 80%, 70%	0	No physical side effects	Unsafe, constant worry if period late	0%
Diaphragm	not widely used by adults or teens	Low	Low occurrence of cervical irritation	Disruption to inter-course decreases chance of use	0%
Vasectomy/ Tubal ligate	99% - not advised for teen use.	High	No physical side effects, no pregnancy	Permanent	0% Theoretically May have transitory depression.

Birth Control: Which Contraceptive Method is Best for You?

Purpose: This exercise attempts to match lifestyles with birth control methods. It should help you and your partner select a method of birth control that you will both feel comfortable using.
Directions: Check **YES** or **NO** for each statement as it applies to you and, if appropriate, your partner.

1) You have a set routine.	YES	NO
2) You prefer a method with no bother.	YES	NO
3) You have a good memory.	YES	NO
4) You are forgetful.	YES	NO
5) You have very heavy, crampy periods.	YES	NO
6) You are a risk-taker.	YES	NO
7) You have sexual intercourse frequently.	YES	NO
8) You need a birth control method right away.	YES	NO
9) You are comfortable with your own sexuality.	YES	NO
10) You dislike doctors and pelvic exams.	YES	NO
11) You are concerned about venereal disease.	YES	NO
12) You have a cooperative partner.	YES	NO
13) You have premature ejaculations.	YES	NO
14) You have patience and a sense of humor.	YES	NO
15) You have sexual intercourse infrequently.	YES	NO
16) You have a lot of privacy.	YES	NO
17) You are a nursing mother.	YES	NO

Scoring: If you answered **YES** to numbers:
1. 1, 3, 5, and 7, then the **birth control pill** might be a good choice.
2. 2, 4, and 6, then **depo-provera** or a **norplant** might be considered.
3. 8, 10, 12, and 14, then **contraceptive foams** might be most appropriate.
4. 9, 11, and 13, then **condom**s might be the best choice.
5. 15, 16, and 17, then consider using a **diaphragm** with **cream** or **jelly.**

Abstinence is the most normal, safe, and effective birth control measure available to teens. However, some teens choose to be sexually active. If your responses indicated there is more than **one method of birth control** for you, remember you can use various methods of birth control throughout your life. This score is not absolute, it is a guide to assist you, your partner, and your health care provider in making the best choice.

QUESTIONS FOR CONSIDERATION:

1)   Given the mobility of our society and surveys that show an increasing rate of sexual activity in the teen years, is it possible that a teen pregnancy is "accidental?"   Comment on this statement as a contributing factor to teen pregnancy.

2)   How does body image relate to the developmental stage of adolescence and teen sexuality?

3)   You are sixty-five years old.   In light of a half-century of changes, what advice would you give today's fifteen-year-old about birth control?

4)   Can a pregnant teen change his or her value system to prevent a second pregnancy? Discuss.

5)   How do family values change one's susceptibility to sexually transmitted diseases?

6)   What organisms and their modes of transmission are fatal to the fetus?

7)   What is certain about a cure for AIDS at this time?

8)   Is hepatitis-B a sexually transmitted disease and is it curable?

9)   Are the causative organisms of AIDS and chlamydia the same the world over?   What implications are there for future treatment of these sexually transmitted diseases?

10) Look at "Sex and the Single Teen" on page 65 to decide which decisions are reversible and which ones are not; which ones are life-threatening, and which are not.

MODULE ELEVEN
HORMONES, HUMOR, AND GOOD GRIEF

"Resiliency"

Diana inched a tiny foot into her bathroom slipper as she sat on the edge of her bed. "If I stand up," she thought, "I can't even see my feet because my stomach is getting so big." Angrily Diana threw on a bathrobe and did not take it off until she had passed the bathroom mirror and was safely in the shower. "The mirror will be steamy so there is no danger of seeing myself after the shower," Diana absentmindedly reckoned to herself.

Diana had a hard time finding jeans and a baggy shirt to wear in her diminishing wardrobe. No one at school really noticed that she was six months pregnant. Diana expanded her baggiest jeans with two safety pins fastened end to end through the top buttonholes. Recently Diana had been expanding the jean waistband with a couple of heavy-duty rubber bands and wearing her largest sweater to cover her hips. The zipper engaged to the midway point. Thankfully the dress code around school didn't demand much more than keeping clean.

No matter, the whole situation was depressing and Diana hoped she wouldn't lose Nick because she was getting "fat," and he had been helping with the doctor bills too! And there was her job, how was she going to keep her pregnancy a secret when she couldn't even reach the counter to hand customers their food. "The Boss must know by now," mused Diana. "Why do I always have to be the one to tell them; why don't they just ask me if I'm pregnant? It would be a lot easier."

The intensity with which a pregnant teen and her partner complain about and react to the woman's changing body image often symbolizes the intensity of their grief over their losses because of the pregnancy. For the first two trimesters there has been an immense amount of planning to do, but there has been little concrete evidence of pregnancy. Body changes signal a need to cope with loss of teen dating and carefree times, loss of relationships with friends who feel uncomfortable about a teen pregnancy, loss of educational and job opportunities, and loss of family if relationships are denied after a teen pregnancy occurs. A teen woman has the greatest fear of losing her partner and the security of love and money that he represents. The teen man who is not committed to his partner finds it convenient to deny fatherhood to the point that he believes it himself.

Imagined losses can be worse than the real losses of teen pregnancy. Not all teen men leave their pregnant partners, particularly if they have support to help them stay. Often teen pregnancy improves family relationships and helps mothers, fathers, sons and daughters form new bonds. Communities and schools too can choose to support and humanize the pregnant teen.

> **GOAL: To process the grief losses of premature teen sexualization assisted by the positive nature of hormones and humor.**

Objective One: Understand gender, pheromones, and degrees of sexualization.

Objective Two: Name each grief loss and state its perspective as an asset instead of a liability.

Objective Three: Understand the stages of grieving and their cyclical repetition as Elizabeth Kubler-Ross applied them to young people.

Objective Four: Raise awareness of family denial and isolation, anger, depression, bargaining, and acceptance that may be progressing at a rate different from that of the teen.

Objective Five: Recognize, acknowledge, and process false signs of good humor that border on hysteria.

METHOD: Clarification about gender identity and sexualization is important. At birth gender identifies a baby. Responses to the infant affirm their "girlness" or "boyness" and the youngster goes on proudly to acknowledge herself or himself as a girl or a boy. This acknowledgment says nothing of sexualization or that passage from childhood to the teenhood that feels and deals with sexual responses.

Our society gives very fuzzy indicators about the "rites of passage" to our teens.

Our society gives very fuzzy indicators to our teens about the "rites of passage." It is possible that they interpret the silence and lack of clarity about sexualization as something negative. Documentation from the health questionnaire shows an avoidance of family discussions about dating and pregnancy among those teens who seek information about birth control outside the family. Seeking help because of teen pregnancy increase a female teen's vulnerability to negative reactions from her family and initiates a cycle of reactions similar to the cycle of grieving described by Elizabeth Kubler-Ross. This cycle of grieving has five stages which Kubler-Ross defined. They are denial and isolation, anger, bargaining, depression, and acceptance. These stages are much less pronounced if a teen is sexualized by his or her own choices to become intimate with a partner and to use birth control. These stages connect the process of sexualization to intense grieving if intercourse has been forced or coerced on either the male or the female. Added confusion and overwhelming grief occur, even to the point of suicide, when sexualization against one's will ends in an untimely pregnancy and cannot be hidden. The issues of grief relating to adoption and abortion are considered further in Module Sixteen, "Other Pregnancy Outcomes."

Negative attitudes are an inescapable part of today's society. Teens share the personal loss of control over their circumstances. Yet these same teens need reminding that they have control over their responses. Distinct positive outcomes develop if we name the concerns of teen sexualization, birth control, and pregnancy and begin to view them as assets. Historically, we have talked about the pregnant girl as the most vulnerable, but nonpregnant couples go through similar cycles of trial and error to establish stable relationships where they will not lose their self-worth.

If we allow ourselves to view teen sexualization in a positive light, the stage is set for problem-solving that gets results. "List your worst problems as a teen. Now, rank these needs and label your worst concern, 'number one.' Next, opposite the concern, imagine the most positive outcome or answer you could have to the problem. Now brainstorm or discuss all the steps you are taking to reach the goal of attaining the positive outcome. Perhaps you cannot find the best solution immediately. Ask yourself, 'What is realistic?' In the everyday world of planning, this is the exact process one uses to solve problems. Begin practicing now, because effective problem-solving will benefit you for life."

The following are some concerns that can have positive outcomes with encouraging results. First, the change in body image is countered by a teen and her partner who become aware of good nutrition and standard mealtimes. Teen mothers listen to encouragement to stop smoking and drinking and, in about eighty percent of situations, voluntarily stop chemical use and abuse while they are pregnant. Teen fathers have a concrete excuse to stop using with their friends and be supportive of their partner's nonuse. Nonuse continues into child-raising if teen partners and their extended families continue to be supportive of positive changes.

Second, teen parents sense a lack of the support from other teens whose present life interests do not include nurturing children. However, the basic maturational issues of all teens are similar. If pregnant and nonpregnant students are taught to be nonjudgmental, they will find that they are all working on dating and relationships and whether or not to be sexually active. They are all concerned about academic commitments so they will have a future that holds good job opportunities. They are all working on separating from their families of origin and becoming independent and self-sufficient; they are all making personal commitments to mature without the effects of drug and alcohol use and abuse.

Third, teens can change difficulty to success in family relationships. Teen parents and their families can use the nine-month time period to discuss the many disappointments of teen pregnancy and seek common ground that makes their love bond stronger. Without the motivation of a teen pregnancy this problem-solving may take much longer. For instance, a common struggle is a decision to support marriage of the teen couple or to discourage the relationship. The intensity of teen pregnancy requires a responsible attitude from the male adolescent. Teen fathers are asked to acknowledge and support their child even if they are not in a continuing relationship with the mother.

By law, teen pregnancy officially emancipates a teen mother and a teen father from the financial support of their family of origin. The choice to be separate from one's family increases the teen's awareness and appreciation of the family that is supportive and caring. Often teen fathers and mothers will not choose welfare because grandparents of the child provide adequate resources. In other cases a pregnancy shows a teen the harsh reality of no one but himself or herself to rely on; in those situations Aid to Families With Dependent Children and the Women, Infants and Children's programs are life-sustaining.

Lastly, the use of humor and a sense of well-being comes naturally to adolescents. The capers of the high school years are a challenge to adults, but teens are a lighthearted inspiration because they "let go" of problems easily. Natural substances found in the body in the form of endorphins and hormones help teens deal with stress.

In the Middle East and the Orient raising large fields of the opium poppy, is legal. This cash crop finds its way to the legal and illicit drug markets of the United States. Doctors prescribe such opiates as codeine, morphine, or demerol to control pain. Heroin and hashish are the illicit "exogenous morphines" taken for increasing the sensation of pleasure. Dr. Arthur Goldstein is the scientist credited with isolating "endogenous morphines" or "endorphins" from receptor sites of the human pituitary gland and the brain. In other words, our body produces opiates of its own that lock into receptor sites in the central nervous system to heighten pleasure and control pain.

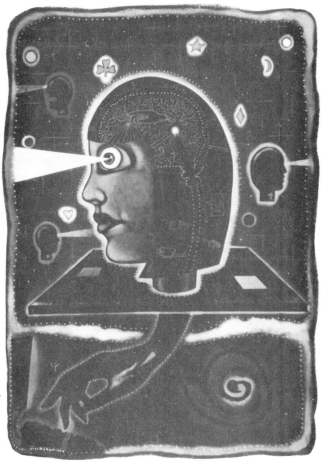

Norman Cousins book, *Anatomy of an Illness* popularized Goldstein's theory. Cousins, an editor for *The Saturday Review*, laughed himself back to health after a life-threatening bout with ankylosing spondylitis. Cousins describes the way laughter healed his mind and body, "I made the joyous discovery that ten minutes of genuine belly laughter had an anesthetic effect and would give me at least two hours of pain free sleep." He would turn on episodes of Candid Camera or old films of the Marx Brothers or have his wife or nurse read to him from such classics as the *Treasury of American Humor*.

The idea of biologist David Berliner that we have natural hormones that exist to give us a sense of well-being is gaining popularity. It is claimed that a gland in our nose responds to chemicals attractants called pheromones. These substances play a part in basic emotions of hunger, fear, and attraction to the opposite sex, because of them we search or "smell" for fulfillment. One would expect that the response of fulfillment would be one of ecstasy or rapture; it is not, rather it a feeling of wholeness, confidence, or well-being. Better understanding of substances such as pheromones may hold a key to the future prevention of teen pregnancy.

Life is an adventure with ups and downs. There are many joys mixed in. We need to watch for and emphasize those joys rather than dwelling on the negative and down times. An expectation of joy, humor, and good personal relationships can come from introspection and participation in group sharing.

QUESTIONS FOR CONSIDERATION:

1)   The societal paradigm of leaving the discussion of sexuality and morality to parents, church, and home may be changing. Is there need for a new paradigm about family values? What are the new concepts in this shift? How will we know whether the new paradigm is more effective than the old?

2)   The idea of dealing with grief by acknowledging stages of change gained acceptance through the work of Elizabeth Kubler-Ross. What is her theory, how is it used, and what meaning does it have for the study of teen sexualization and teen pregnancy prevention?

3)   Find the law concerning teen emancipation and pregnancy?   What if a child is born? Examine and discuss the legal effects of this law.

4)   As a facilitator, how would one increase the use of humor?

5)   What types of humor and what humorous authors are popular among teenagers today? Include musicians in your search.

6)   Does laughter always show humor? Consider uncontrollable laughter that borders on hysteria, plus smiling constantly and laughing nervously to cover pain.

7)   Does the manufacture of perfume already utilize David Berliner's ideas without knowing the exact chemical significance of attractants?

8)   Give examples of the anger that teens and their parents express through the months of acknowledging a pregnancy and years of parenting the child.

9)   Is the stage of denial of teen pregnancy great enough that a teen father begins to believe that he is not a father? How does a teen mother deal with that same degree of denial and grieving when she has the physical evidence of pregnancy?

10) Are there employers in your community who are empathetic to the job needs of teens? Does this empathy extend to the pregnant and parenting teen? What community agency helps train and find employment for teens who have children?

MODULE TWELVE
GESTATION, LABOR AND DELIVERY, PRE-TERM LABOR

"A Universal Language"

The loose windows rattled in the door as three small people pounded desperately to rouse our attention. Stumbling down the steps, the troika pulled me along until I was running with them down a dusty path beyond the confines of our neighborhood. My husband and I had been in Lashkar Gah, Afghanistan, for two months as Peace Corps volunteers. The only Afghan families we had met were in our neighborhood.

Upon opening their compound door, the youngsters led me through a garden to an adobe hut where a young pregnant woman, presumably their mother, lay groaning on a *toshak* or mattress in the corner of the room. "*Modar?*" I questioned, pointing to the woman on the *toshak*. "*Neh,*" the young people clicked their tongues, "No" in chorus, and the middle girl offered, "It is our aunt, please help us?" with an inflection at the end of the command as if it were a question.

I stationed the two younger girls by their aunt's side while the oldest one and I hurried back to my compound to gather rubber gloves, basins, clips, and towels. Less than an hour later, Mahtub delivered a stillborn baby boy of five months gestation with the amniotic sac still intact. She lamented to Allah in a singsong moan because the claws of fate had grabbed her male baby, a precious progenitor.

> . . . birthing infants was as universal as smiles or a musical refrain; its positive quality had been there from the dawn of time and I didn't even have to speak.

My Persian was broken and difficult to understand. Yet as I began to get other requests to be a midwife to the neighborhood women, I realized that birthing infants was as universal as smiles or a musical refrain; its positive quality had been there from the dawn of time and I didn't even have to speak. However, if a girl was born, I would offer, "*Allah, shakor,*" to thank God for a baby girl. The Afghan women offered thanks to Allah only when a male child was born.

By the time we left Afghanistan, I had delivered over a dozen babies, the oldest of whom was Sahrina. My parting memory of our Lashkar Gah neighborhood is of Sahrina sitting on our compound steps in her little pink plastic shoes waving at our truck as it pulled away from a home, a family, and a neighborhood that had sustained us for two years.

PART ONE: GESTATION

GOAL: To visualize conception and growth of the fetus through books, videos, models, and group discussion.

Objective One: Learn the terms of reproduction and gestation.

Objective Two: Review the anatomy and physiology of the reproductive system.

Objective Three: Review the concept of menstruation and see the control that the pituitary gland and hormones have on ovulation, sperm production, and fertilization.

Objective Four: Trace the path of the ovum, the sperm, and the zygote, and the zygote's implantation into the uterus.

Objective Five: Understand fetal growth from conception to full-term gestation.

Objective Six: Introduce the variety of factors that can interrupt full-term gestation.

METHOD: Multimedia resources highlight gestation in a way that promotes teen interest, understanding, and discussion of pregnancy. We teach the vocabulary of gestation first. *Pregnancy, Day By Day*, a book that highlights the daily progress of pregnancy is interesting to the teen who has a family member who is pregnant or to the teen couple who is pregnant A "Glossary of Reproductive Anatomy and Related Terms" is provided on page 104.

The anatomy and physiology of the reproductive system requires review. Use the *Birth Atlas, A Child Is Born* and Dr. Robert Bradley's video "Gestation" for basic information. Nova's video highlighted by the photography of Lennard Nilsson entitled the "Miracle of Life" is an hour in length and is valuable to build on a basic understanding of gestation. An expanded resource list is found in the "References" for Module Twelve on page 109.

In any culture, the intrinsic factors that control outcomes of gestation are inheritance and maternal health. Extrinsic factors that generate irregular outcomes to pregnancy are induced termination of pregnancy and environmental and ingested toxins. This module would not be complete without discussing natural and induced complications to teen pregnancy. The handout, "Common Tests During Pregnancy," provided on page 79, underscores the need for early pregnancy confirmation. "Risk Factors In Fetal Development" on page 51 takes into account the damaging characteristics of alcohol, tobacco, and other drugs (ATOD). Module Eight's focus is entirely on the issue of alcohol, tobacco, and other drugs.

PART TWO: LABOR AND DELIVERY

GOAL: To address teen fear of labor and delivery and encourage healthy anticipation.

Objective One: Review the anatomy and physiology of reproduction in a way that characterizes birth as a happy event.

Objective Two: Understand the significance of birth to a teen, her partner, and the grandparents.

Objective Three: Acknowledge monthly pregnancy changes that may be annoying but normal.

Objective Four: Advertise and promote prepared childbirth classes.

Objective Five: Arrange for a tour of the birthing room and the nursery.

METHOD: This module illustrates interdependence on community resources. Review anatomy and physiology of birthing. For group work that serves pregnant teens and their partners, invite a guest speaker who will direct pregnant teens to the most helpful classes on coached childbirth. Special arrangements often include two four-hour Saturday teen sessions with a tour of the birthing rooms to alleviate anxiety for teens who are near delivery.

During each pregnancy, concerns for such conditions as round ligament pain and Braxton-Hicks contractions arise. It is important to acknowledge these normal but annoying distractions of pregnancy. Reading material and group time with students who have experienced delivery are good sources of support.

PART THREE: PRETERM LABOR

GOAL: To acknowledge preterm emergencies without promoting fear.

Objective One: Educate teens about increased pregnancy risks correlated with adolescence.

Objective Two: Encourage early prenatal medical care to reduce risks of preterm delivery in the pregnant teen.

Objective Three: Review adequate prenatal care as a measure to prevent emergencies.

Objective Four: Discuss the importance of informing teachers and counselors about a teen pregnancy because of preterm pregnancy risks in the classroom.

Objective Five: Initiate discussion with the grandparents and partners about preterm labor and emergencies and enlist their help.

METHOD: Adolescent pregnancy carries greater risk of miscarriage and premature delivery than does adult pregnancy. Early medical care will prevent problems. Normal measures such as urine and blood testing and nutritional counseling is a part of routine prenatal checkups to ensure healthy gestation. A good system of communication can reduce anxiety and avert a problem.

In school, teachers, administrators, nurses, and counselors need to know about a student pregnancy because having a classroom emergency as early as the third month is possible. Teens must give written permission for this exchange of information. Reviewing signs of preterm labor and false labor can be done with parents, partners, teachers, and counselors. These signs include the following: 1) low back pain that is constant and does not improve with rest and relaxation, 2) clear vaginal discharge that increases with movement, 3) lower abdominal cramps that are similar to menstrual cramps, but increase in intensity and duration, and 4) bloody vaginal discharge. If there are fears of any kind, call the physician, a health care professional, or the hospital emergency room to avoid endangering mother and child. The "References" for Module Twelve list other sources of information about preterm labor.

Common Tests During Pregnancy

Trimester I - Fetus is 0-12 weeks gestation and up to 1inch in length and 3/4 ounces in weight.

1. Pregnancy Tests - Urine and blood tests of hormone HCG within the first month of pregnancy will detect pregnancy with 97% accuracy.

2. Rh Factor - A negative blood type is not as common as a positive one; if both mother and baby are Rh negative there will be no problem. If mother and baby have different Rh factors, a substance to prevent problems with the baby's blood antigen reaction is given.

3. VDRL Blood Test - A test to detect the bacteria that cause the sexually transmitted disease of syphilis. Antibodies to the disease are given so the baby does not contract syphilis. Vaginal and blood cultures are done if symptoms of other STDs exist.

4. Complete Blood Counts - A blood test done each trimester to see that proper nutrients are present in quantities adequate for normal fetal growth and development.

5. Urine Test - The urine is tested for abnormal amounts of protein and sugar. Urine sugar can indicate diabetes; urine protein and high blood pressure can indicate toxemia.

6. Rubella Titer - A blood test to show that maternal rubella antibodies are present. If the titer is low, the pregnant woman needs to avoid ill children and adults who are complaining of flu symptoms and neck aches. Rubella, if contracted during pregnancy, can cause blindness, deafness, mental retardation, or heart defects in the unborn child.

7. Fasting blood sugar - A blood test to detect sugar-related diabetes is done if sugar was found on urinalysis. If the fasting blood sugar is positive, then a glucose tolerance test will be done in the second trimester. Early detection may require induced labor or Caesarean section to reduce maternal and child complications.

Trimester II - Fetus is 13-26 weeks gestation and up to 2 pounds in weight, 1 foot long.

1. Alpha fetoprotein (AFP) - A blood test usually done before 16 weeks gestation to *screen* for some types of birth defects. If it is positive, it does *not* mean that a birth defect exists; it only indicates that further testing should be done.

2. Ultrasound - A living sonogram of the fetus most commonly done to check for low birth weight or fetal failure to thrive, twins, amount of amniotic fluid, or size of a baby before a Caesarean section.

Trimester III - Fetus is 27 - 40 weeks (full-term) gestation and up to 7 pounds, 21 inches long.

The health care provider repeats tests as deemed necessary.

QUESTIONS FOR CONSIDERATION:

1) Use new terms to write a paragraph describing a phase of gestation.

2) Describe Dr. Bradley's role in the interactive development of natural childbirth and coached childbirth.

3) Describe ten common annoyances of pregnancy and their remedies.

4) Investigate and make a directory of phone numbers of community resources that are helpful in dealing with issues of labor and delivery. Which of these agencies are most helpful to teens?

5) What factors contribute to miscarriage or preterm labor and delivery in the adolescent? How can these outcomes be avoided?

6) Who has the legal right to know about a teen pregnancy?

7) Interview an obstetrician, a physician's assistant, a nurse or a nurse practitioner regarding preterm labor and delivery among their adolescent clients.

8) Discuss effective ways of teaching teen fathers to be helpful during labor and delivery.

9) Interview a physician about the cost of labor and delivery. Which tests are routine and included in the price of the basic clinical visit and which tests and procedures are considered special and of added cost?

10) What public health facilities and financial assistance are available to promote healthy pregnancies?

MODULE THIRTEEN
NUTRITION

"The Adage"

Our community held a birthday party today to honor those who, for twenty years, had helped feed countless women, infants, and children in need.

The Town Council and the City Manager were there. The Mayor gave a speech and said she had been visited by angels; we all nodded and applauded and sang.

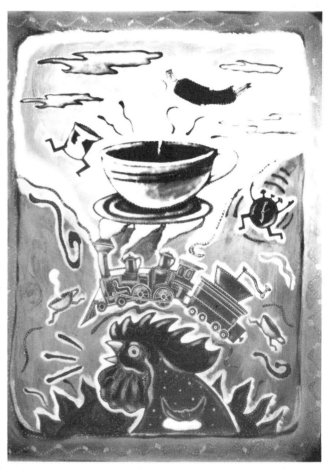

Noted leaders and ministers were in the audience from the Friendship Circle for we have not wiped out violence and battering within families. They do healing when there is a gathering.

Our local AAUP came because they are wealthy and wise and had mass-produced a warm, colorful sweatshirt on which they inscribed a motto over the round, happy faces of our children. "For it is time," they said, " to revive the ancient adage proclaiming, 'It takes a village to raise a child.'"

Summit People were there because we are a mountain people and pay homage to God who protects us in our isolated province. They closed with a Collect passed to us from the Sioux, *"Great Spirit, Great Spirit, my Grandfather, all over the Earth living things are all alike. Look upon the faces of children without number and with children in their arms, that they may face the winds and walk the good road to the day of quiet."*

GOAL: To apply the precepts of the American Dietetics Association to educating teens about good nutrition and its relation to sexuality.

Objective One: Teach good nutrition using The Food Pyramid.

Objective Two: Explore information about nutrition by inviting a speaker from Women, Infants, and Children.

Objective Three: Use a diet recall form to assess the nutritional level of each teen and to teach to the points of that assessment.

Objective Four: Foster teen self-responsibility for nutrition.

Objective Five: Rely on outside agencies and private physicians to investigate a teen's nutritional risks using blood and urine glucose tolerance testing for sugar metabolism, urine testing for ketosis, and ultrasound testing for fetal size in the pregnant teen.

METHOD: Balanced nutrition and adequate rest promote good adolescent health. Providing education about adequate nutrition is one way a village can raise the collective well-being of its young people. The undernutrition of our adolescent population is as frightening as their use and abuse of alcohol, tobacco, and other drugs. In the book, *Treating Bulimia*, authors Weiss, Katzman, and Wolchik assert that the true mental obsession of the eating disordered person and the alcoholic is not food or drink, but the approval of another person. This same mental attitude, that of pleasing another person to feel fulfilled, may be an underlying factor in teen pregnancy as well.

In the module on the genogram, we discussed the ordinal positions of family members. Although the "hero," the "lost child," or the "mascot" of a dysfunctional family system may become pregnant it is most common to see the "scapegoat" of the family deal with unintended pregnancy. The ability to pull the family together over a crisis affirms identity and pregnancy becomes the issue a family cannot deny; pregnancy also becomes the instrument to heal broken bonds and make a teen feel that they are part of the family.

Nutrition, as the focus of change, is a nonthreatening way to acquaint oneself with the daily health of any teen, pregnant or not. The "Personal Diet Recall Guide" on page 84 helps initiate this discussion. When a teen is referred to the school counselor or the school nurse for nutritional needs, a record of daily activities, including eating patterns, needs assessing. With help, the adolescent recalls and records eating patterns. The guide has a column of suggested foods for healthy nutrition. This is followed by seven columns to record food intake on a daily basis for one week or less. There are five rows. The first four ask for breakfast, lunch, dinner, and snack recall. The final row contains spaces to mark the number of daily servings in each food category that is a minimum daily requirement.

Ask the student to continue recording, not changing, eating patterns for a week. Then ask for a repeat appointment after recording food intake and eating patterns. If nutrition is poor, discuss what small changes can be initiated to give a teen power over his or her nutrition and improve how they feel. Fact sheets and three dimensional pyramid models patterned after the information on page 85 are available from the American Dietetics Association or the United States Department of Agriculture as adjunct teaching tools to the recall guide.

The nutrition module introduces the self-care tasks of a pregnant teen in a nonthreatening manner. Because fetal health is important from the beginning of gestation, early nutritional assessment is important if pregnancy is suspected. Repeated discussions about the food pyramid and use of the recall guide to assess nutritional status and self-responsibility is repeated monthly. Vitamins and other dietary supplements taken during pregnancy introduce the idea of caring for the new life even before delivery.

This module shows interdependence on other community agencies as well. First, the private physician provides information on nutrition. Second, if the doctor notes a need for further assistance, the help of a hospital nutrition center or a home health agency is recruited. Home health pregnancy services are authorized to make home visits and become effective as they report findings to the family, the private physician, and the school nurse or counselor.

A third agency, Women, Infants and Children, called WIC, is helpful when household finances are short and there is need of food to supplement nutrition. A broad spectrum of educational services is available through the local and state public health departments on referral from the WIC project.

Personal Diet Recall Guide

Name:_____   Weekly Recall Dates: _____to_____

Dairy Group 2-3 servings milk, yogurt cheese, ice cream	Breakfast	Breakfast	Breakfast	Breakfast	Breakfast	Breakfast	Breakfast
Fruit Group 2-4 servings canned, raw Vegetable 3-5 servings cooked, raw	Lunch	Lunch	Lunch	Lunch	Lunch	Lunch	Lunch
Bread Group 6-11 servings bread, pasta rice, cereal	Dinner	Dinner	Dinner	Dinner	Dinner	Dinner	Dinner
Meat Group Meat Sub 2-3 servings lean meat, fish, poultry, eggs legumes	Snacks	Snacks	Snacks	Snacks	Snacks	Snacks	Snacks
Adolescent minimum requirement =	Milk 0000 Fruit 000 Veg 000 Bread 000 Meat 000 Meat Sub 0	Milk 0000 Fruit 000 Veg 000 Bread 000 Meat 000 Meat Sub 0	Milk 0000 Fruit 000 Veg 000 Bread 000 Meat 000 Meat Sub 0	Milk 0000 Fruit 000 Veg 000 Bread 000 Meat 000 Meat Sub 0	Milk 0000 Fruit 000 Veg 000 Bread 000 Meat 000 Meat Sub 0	Milk 0000 Fruit 000 Veg 000 Bread 000 Meat 000 Meat Sub 0	Milk 0000 Fruit 000 Veg 000 Bread 000 Meat 000 Meat Sub 0

The Food Guide Pyramid

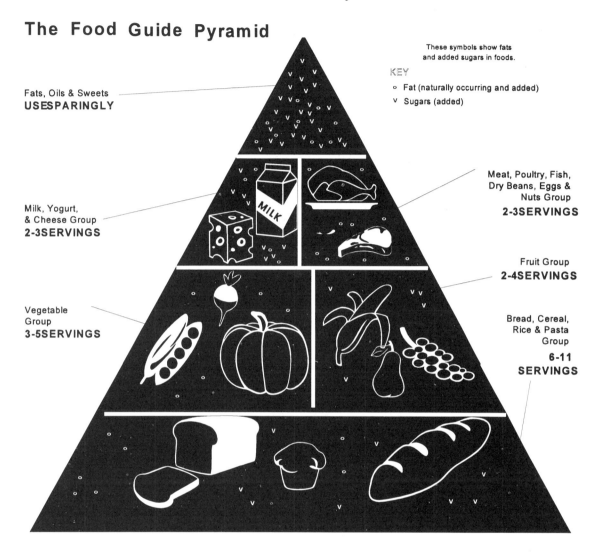

The Food Guide Pyramid

These symbols show fats and added sugars in foods.

KEY
o Fat (naturally occurring and added)
v Sugars (added)

Fats, Oils & Sweets
USE SPARINGLY

Milk, Yogurt,
& Cheese Group
2-3 SERVINGS

Meat, Poultry, Fish,
Dry Beans, Eggs &
Nuts Group
2-3 SERVINGS

Fruit Group
2-4 SERVINGS

Vegetable
Group
3-5 SERVINGS

Bread, Cereal,
Rice & Pasta
Group
**6-11
SERVINGS**

The United States Department of Agriculture has devised a way to make choosing a healthy diet easy. The USDA recently released a revised Food Guide Pyramid. It provides dietary guidance for Americans two years of age and older. The primary message is to eat a variety of foods from all the group in moderate amounts. Additionally, the Pyramid focuses on reducing the amount of fat and sugar in the diet and increasing the intake of fiber and water.

Different people have different needs; the Pyramid gives a range for numbers of servings of each type of food. The number of servings can also vary according to the age, sex, size, and activity level of the individual. Everyone should have at least the minimum number of servings in each category.

QUESTIONS FOR CONSIDERATION:

1)   The food pyramid is a new ADA-recommended teaching device. What nutritional developments precipitated these recent changes in the study of nutrition?

2)   How can monitoring blood pressure and discussing information from the Personal Diet Recall Guide complement each other in nutrition counseling of an overweight teen?

3)   How does the Personal Diet Recall Guide help nonpregnant and pregnant teens establish self-responsibility for nutrition?

4)   If the federally funded Women, Infants, and Children program is reduced, are there local and state sources to support good nutrition?

5)   Family patterns of addiction influence teen nutrition. Give two examples of addiction that impact teen nutrition.

6)   If a teen who is practicing anorexia or bulimia becomes pregnant, how is determination made about the reason for a missed period?

7)   Is there medical evidence of a correlation between rising numbers of adolescent diabetics and adult malnutrition due to alcohol abuse?

8)   Will welfare reform endanger nutritional health care delivery to the undernourished adolescent?

9)   What would you do if you expected false reporting on a diet recall assignment?

10) How is malnourishment of the fetus evident to the physician?

MODULE FOURTEEN
MALE RESPONSIBILITY, FATHER BONDING

"Sean's Story"

In his book, *The Moral Animal*, author Robert Wright details the growth of a phenomenon called evolutionary psychology. Wright explores the fine-tuned mating dance of the Stone Age man and woman and shows how they can trace the characteristics of masculine and feminine sexuality to the dawn of mankind. William Allman writes about the work of Wright and psychologist, David Buss in "The Mating Game," and says, "A woman has no doubt that she is the mother of her children. For a man, however, paternity is never more than conjecture, and so men have evolved psychologies with a heightened concern about a mate's infidelity. Since women make the greater biological investment in offspring, their psychologies are more concerned about a mate's reneging on his commitment, and, therefore, they are more attentive to signs that their mates might be attaching themselves emotionally to other women."

Whether these theorists are correct or not, there are examples within the patterns of teen dating, commitment, and child care that illustrate this conjecture about paternity. However, another science is authenticating paternity. It is the technology that identifies a baby's origins by the deoxyribonucleic acid that marks his or her cell structure, called DNA testing.

How a young man views his paternity undergoes many changes during the pregnancy. When a baby is born, the reality of being a "daddy" becomes more concrete. Today teen dads continue to view their child care responsibilities differently than teen moms do. For that reason, I will let Sean tell his own story. You have already met his partner, Kate, in an earlier vignette.

Cars were my life. I don't like kids and never imaged myself the father of a kid. In my figuring, they were just little rug rats who took my tools when I was under my hood trying to fix an engine.

Then Kate, this one girl who I sorta liked, always used to babysit my little brother. Anyway, she was always around 'cause they lived next door. In those days her dad used to holler out the window at the "damn kids" and I sorta felt sorry for Kate.

Then one day he left, Kate's Dad I mean, and her mom was gone all the time too. One thing led to another and before I knew it, Kate said she was seeing me, and then we were going out, and then Kate got pregnant.

I felt like bashing a wall in all the time last year, and I dropped out of school to work on my cars. Then Tracy Jereen was born. We both really like her. I don't live with Kate and I don't ever want to, but watch out Madonna, my Tracy is a looker already. I'll always be her dad and watch out if anybody lays a hand on her.

> **GOAL: To acknowledge the lifelong responsibility of a father to his child and to encourage a lasting bond and a permanent attachment.**

Objective One: Raise awareness of teen males to sexual responsibility.

Objective Two: Address the denial of fatherhood.

Objective Three: Invite male involvement as father of the baby and partner of the teen mother.

Objective Four: Encourage a teen father to be a part of a support group; make provisions for a weekly guest pass if the father is beyond high school age.

Objective Five: Raise awareness of the legal and financial responsibilities of parenting.

METHOD: An appeal from the women of single-parent families is gaining attention as they make monetary demands on the men who have abandoned their children. These women are a living statistic as the number of children in families with only a mother grew from 5.1 million in 1960 to 15.6 million by 1993. See "Current Statistics" on page 114.

Former U.S. Attorney General William Barr said, "If you look at the one factor that most closely correlates with crime, it's not poverty, it's not the lack of employment, it's not poor education. It's the absence of the father in the family." We as a nation in crisis listen intently to the mothers when the rising crime rate impacts our lives and our pocketbooks.

> **Former U.S. Attorney General William Barr said, "If you look at the one factor that most closely correlates with crime, it's not poverty, it's not the lack of employment, it's not poor education. It's the absence of the father in the family."**

The mere presence of a parenting teen father makes a sobering impression on teen males who are not pregnant or parenting. Yet this person-to-person method of educating teens about the perils of teen fathering is not used often enough. Supporting teen fathers does not promote or demote the idea of marriage. No matter what the status of the couple's relationship becomes, it is important that the connection of the father to his child be initiated and nurtured. When episodes of denial of paternity occur, counseling support is necessary with recognition that denial is a part of grieving experienced by the male teen at the loss of his freedom.

The pediatric research of A.B. Elsters and Frank F. Furstenberg in the last decade come to similar conclusions about the value of father-child bonding. Generalization about this bonding and attachment is fourfold: 1) it strengthens the identities of the child and the teen father, 2) the child responds with attachment and does not experience abandonment, 3) the need for support becomes concrete because the father feels needed, and 4) financial responsibilities are acknowledged as a part of bearing and raising a child. The work of Elsters and Furstenberg lay a foundation for a kinder and gentler way to rock the cradle of father-child relationships.

The goal of a young organization called National Fatherhood Initiative says, "Reinstating fatherhood as a national priority will be accomplished one child and one neighborhood at a time." At a recent conference on building youth and families, Dr. Wade Horn, Director of National Fatherhood Initiative, cited the efforts of men like Bill Stephney, President of StepSun Music to team with NFI and penetrate the world of entertainment with messages about responsible fatherhood.

Dr. Horn further cited the work of a dedicated man who is "accomplishing the reinstatement of fatherhood one child at a time." This man has a network to find new fathers and encourage immediate visits to their infants. The attachment and bonding of the first visits tie men to their children in a way that no amount of scorn and legal retribution can. The National Fatherhood Initiative is a source of brochures and information to men and women who want to expand their knowledge and application of parenting skills.

Social service centers provide information and support to mothers and fathers who need financial help to raise a child. In teen pregnancies, it is usually the woman who remains the custodial parent. If she receives any form of welfare assistance, most states have child support enforcement provisions to collect support monies from the noncustodial parent. Guest speakers can cover such topics as DNA testing, what to do about the reluctant parent, and legal aspects of demanding child support from the noncustodial parent; however, this can never be a substitute for the love and personal commitment of a caring father or mother.

QUESTIONS FOR CONSIDERATION:

1)   How closely do trends in sexuality among teens mirror the trends of adults? Of the media?

2)   What practical appeal would serve as a deterrent to teen fatherhood in your setting?

3)   Talk about the anger and denial of teen fatherhood as part of the grieving process.

4)   Discuss changes of group dynamic when teen fathers become part of a co-ed support group.

5)   How do the concerns of teen fathers differ from those of teen mothers?

6)   What are the logistics in your setting of admitting the older partner of a pregnant teen to support group?

7)   A quotation from Health and Human Services Secretary, Louis W. Sullivan, states, "The mortality rate of infants born to college-educated but unmarried mothers is higher than for infants born to married high school dropouts." Study the facts behind this quotation and decide if a high school education should continue to be a priority for pregnant and parenting teens. Why or why not?

8)   Does an infant feel the loss of a father even if he or she seems too young to know loss?

9)   Is Murphy Brown's portrayal of unmarried motherhood a myth? Fact: Labor Department statistics show that 44 percent of births to poor white mothers are outside marriage, compared with only 6 percent for white women above the poverty line.

10) "Children are the fastest growing segment of the crime population in the United States." What does this say about the need for involvement of fathers in the lives of their children?

MODULE FIFTEEN
PREPARING FOR CHILD CARE

"Time Banking"

Time is an abstract commodity that does not have boundaries of class or culture. It symbolizes fairness because we all have twenty-four hours to spend daily. The concept of time banking for time conservation is valuable in preparation for coping with child rearing.

For high school students, a structured amount of time is committed to attending school. For activity time coupons or coins are required. Because there are one-hundred and thirty-eight hours in a week, that is the number of coupons needed. The students pair and discuss the general categories of time budgeting, such as, shopping, meal planning and preparation, child care, sleep, beauty and hygiene, homework, school, relaxation, family fun, jobs, and "hanging out."

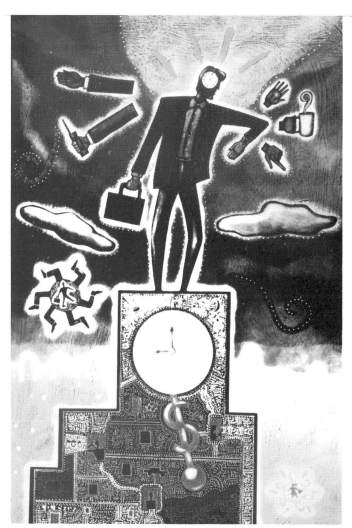

Envelopes receive the coins or coupons as each hour or block of hours is spent. Reporting of activities and outcomes are done at the end of a week's time. Early in pregnancy the perception of responsibility to a baby is unrealistic. Use this exercise individually when a teen is having a difficult time choosing adoption or keeping the baby.

Do a reality check by repeating the time banking activity about two months after a baby is born. A panel presentation by teen parents to nonpregnant students is an effective birth control measure. Pregnant and parenting teens are usually eager to share the changes that have taken place in their perception of child care management after they have become parents. The time banking activity can be used to bring reality to the concerns of child rearing.

GOAL: To help teens recognize the sacrifice of time and commitment of self to responsible child care.

Objective One: Understand the idea of time banking.

Objective Two: Investigate objects and concepts that deter teen pregnancy.

Objective Three: Present financial realities of child care.

Objective Four: Visit and collect information about independent child care homes and centers, private and public health services, and government welfare such as Aid To Families With Dependent Children (AFDC).

Objective Five: Guide students through class scheduling and encourage participation in education that addresses child development and adult living skills.

METHOD: The concept of time banking illustrates the value of spending time wisely in preparing for the commitment to a child. To repeat this exercise sometime after the birth of the baby is enlightening. It is valuable to use this exercise for nonpregnant teens before a parenting teen speaks to them about the realities of child-rearing.

Creative parent minds are constantly at work to deter their teens from an unintended pregnancy. Recently a teen couple, who thought it would be "neat" to have a baby, were asked by their parents to take Elmo, the Sesame Street character, into twenty-four hour tutelage. Smart, those parents! At last report, the teen couple are going their separate ways and Elmo is as happy sitting in a corner as he ever was. "Egg babies" and "Baby-Think-It-Over" graphically communicate the same concept. These gimmicks are used to raise awareness of the infant who needs care, safety, food, diapers, and support twenty-four hours a day whether they are crying, cooing, sleeping, or rappelling the front of the refrigerator.

The primary responsibility of group work before the teen moves to programs that teach parenting skills is to raise awareness of community support resources. Private physicians, public health agencies, and family planning agencies offer monthly appointments to maintain good maternal and infant health and prevent a second teen pregnancy. Private physicians have been known to offer "scholarships" that provide extended birth control in the form of norplant or depoprovera protection. Service organizations donate funds or in-kind services or materials to help parents.

Young parent programs may be provided jointly by the school and the community. Investigation of welfare for teen parents who have no family support is offered. Other innovative programs include the concept of mentoring. Teachers have pledged significant roles of support to students in high school. A program called Mother-To-Mother enlists the help of experienced adult parents to model responsible child-rearing practices to their teen counterparts. Curricular offerings in the high school home economics department include classes in child development, nutrition, and adult living skills. Group work can augment these classes and oversee class scheduling so teen parents are aware of the availability of education that meets their needs.

QUESTIONS FOR CONSIDERATION:

1)   Prepare a plan to deter teen pregnancy by presenting information on "egg babies," "Baby-Think-It-Over," and "bag-of-potato-babies."

2)   Interview a parent and a pastor for innovative ideas to deter teen pregnancy.

3)   Are teen girls more developmentally ready for pregnancy than teen boys?

4)   Use the time banking exercise to help a teen couple look at the pros and cons of adoption.

5)   In advising teen parents about the wise use of time, which areas need emphasis; which areas could be compromised for lack of time?

6)   Does the lack of good time management foster neglect of a baby? What could be done to address this problem?

7)   Investigate the availability of child care in your community. What care is available, what is not? How is the situation remedied?

8)   How do day care budgets meet the individual needs of babies?

9)   Explore other agencies that support teen parents. Check names such as Community Training Institute; Women, Infants, and Children; First Steps; Families First; or other community networks.

10) Most child care centers do not allow ill child attendance. What are the guidelines for declaring an infant ill and unable to attend day care? Where do these children go if their parents are teenagers and need to attend school?

MODULE SIXTEEN
OTHER PREGNANCY OUTCOMES

"Legacy"

We are aware of the poignant joys and harsh realities of teen sexuality and how the extremity of these joys and realities are present in teen pregnancy and parenting. In fairness to pregnant teens and their families, the options of adoption and abortion are also a reality. Making decisions for pregnant teens and their families is not the role of a person outside the family circle. However, giving tools, time, resources, and support to the decision-making process that occurs with teen pregnancy is helpful.

A new approach has tempered the finality of adoption in the past fifteen years. It is called open adoption. Open adoption, as defined by Jeanne Warren Lindsay, in her book *Open Adoption: A Caring Option*, is where, "Birth parents choose adoptive parents for their babies. Adoptive parents may stay in contact with their child's birth parents as facilitated by state or private adoption agencies." Teens often wait until the last trimester of pregnancy to begin counseling and decision-making in this area. In other words, by avoidance, they have bypassed the choice of abortion. The teens can choose any variation of adoption on the open/closed adoption continuum. Open adoption may be the popular choice, but it does not mean that the teens need to choose this option. This poem, author unknown, shows the intense emotional quality of adoption.

Legacy of an Adopted Child

Once there were two women, who never knew each other;
    One you do not remember, the other you call mother.
Two different lives, shaped to make yours one,
    One became your guiding star, the other became your sun.

The first gave you life, and the second taught you how to live it;
    The first gave you a need for love, the second was there to give it.
One gave you a nationality, the other gave you a name;
    One gave you the seed of talent, the other gave you an aim.

One gave you emotions, the other calmed your fears;
    One saw your first sweet smile, the other dried your tears.
One gave you up - that was all that she could do!
    The other prayed for a child, and God led her straight to you.

And now you ask me, through your tears,
    The age-old question through the years.
Heredity or the environment, which are you a product of?
    Neither, my darling - neither, just two different kinds of love.

Author Unknown

Kathleen Silber and Phylis Speedlin have co-authored several editions of *Dear Birthmother*. Their candid and reality-based account of the evolution of open adoption is informative and contains helpful direction in making choices about pregnancy outcomes.

Abortion is the other choice that deserves discussion. As Therese Rondo says in her book, *Grief, Death, and Dying*, we as Americans have a societal myth that grieving, death, and dying are more the issues of the aged than of the young. Discussions about the issues of adolescent loss, that is, teen death due to suicide, disease, or accident goes unacknowledged. Two other authors, Marion Kaczmarek and Barbara Backlund, declare that because of this societal blindness, teen pain at the loss of a romantic partner is rarely considered a loss. If we were to put teen losses on a continuum, grieving the loss resulting from an induced adolescent abortion is so disenfranchised or unacknowledged that our society denies that teens experience grief loss in this area.

This admission puts us in a dilemma. We have already discussed Erik Erikson's theories about the maturational tasks of teens, those of intimacy and independence. To be able to have intimate relationships and to be mature enough to become independent one needs healthy emotional and reasoning faculties. Therein lies our dilemma, and I say "ours" because we as a society strongly influence, by our polity or our silence, the decisions of teens and their families in the tender area of induced abortion.

Numbness assuages the teen grief that comes in the aftermath of induced abortion. Anesthetizing oneself against the emotional aspects of post-abortion grief is the most common teen reaction. Without realizing it, parents affirm numbness because they do not want to see their child in pain. Boyfriends, sometimes approve of numbness and are more likely to keep dating a young woman if she agrees to end the pregnancy and appear obliging about it. When people in the girl's life act out the repression they are feeling, the young woman is not likely to admit her true feelings; she may even avoid contact with clergy or counsel who would remind her of the issue she is trying to forget.

D. E. Balk in his book, *Death Studies*, says, "A counselor's ability to recognize and help an adolescent process grief may determine the adolescent's future capacity to move into an adult stage of dealing with emotions and making decisions." When Balk discusses the recognition and use of an adolescent's religion in aiding the grief process, he says, "Findings show religious belief did not make coping necessarily any easier for teenagers, but the mourning permitted by religion allowed acceptance of death more easily."

A young woman fares better if she has been the primary person to choose abortion. Post-abortion counseling for the teen and her partner is appropriate. Coping skills are actualized and of help in acknowledging the grief, processing it, and then going on with one's life. Whatever the life choice in teen sexuality, it demands the best values that we as a society have to offer.

GOAL: To nonjudgmentally educate pregnant teens about their choices regarding pregnancy outcomes.

Objective One: Realize the importance of time, objectivity, and nonjudgmental attitudes in supporting the pregnant teen.

Objective Two: Support the teens while they rely on peers, parents, clergy, and significant others for decision-making.

Objective Three: Educate the pregnant teen about school and other community resources that aid and support decision-making.

Objective Four: Have names of qualified and competent counseling services available.

METHOD: The decision for keeping the baby, relinquishing the newborn, or aborting the pregnancy is the choice of the pregnant teens and their families. At times when a teen is scared about pregnancy, their first choice of support may be another teen, a teacher, a nurse, a counselor, or a family pastor. In the role of educator and supportive listener, it is a legal obligation to allow teens the time to decide. Because they are at a developmental crossroad coupled with a crisis, supporting a good relationship with their families is important. However, by law, becoming pregnant and bearing a child emancipates a teen from their parents.

There are no easy choices. A supporter's role as an educator is key. Private physicians, clergy, the community agencies of Family Planning, Planned Parenthood, the local hospital, local churches and Mental Health Services are good sources for ideas about available choices. Catholic Social Services provide counseling that supports choice-making. If adoption becomes a possibility, they present a continuum of adoption services from privately handled open adoption to a confidential closed adoption.

Planned Parenthood, Family Planning, and private physicians have information about abortion, its cost, clinics available for services, and access to the confidential counseling that is so important preceding and after an abortion. These agencies and physicians' offices have nurses, nurse practitioners, nurse midwives, and physician assistants who have information about abortion and birth control follow-up.

Abortions are more secret and most teens are not comfortable with group work until they have made a choice. Group participants only support a decision that is already made. Although group support appears more available to teens who are relinquishing their child for adoption or keeping their baby, there *is* care and concern for the young people who choose abortion.

QUESTIONS FOR CONSIDERATION:

1)   Do counselors or other health professionals make decisions about pregnancy outcomes for teens and their families?

2)   Has the new option of open adoption made choices of pregnancy outcomes any easier for the pregnant teen?

3)   List phone numbers and addresses of current contacts who would be helpful in decision-making regarding the outcomes of teen pregnancy.

4)   Many agencies are open during business hours only. How does one handle appointments for pregnant teens who have not disclosed the pregnancy to their parents, are expected to be in school, yet need to make a decision based on investigation of all information available in the community?

5)   Are grieving, death, and dying more the concerns of the old than the young?

6)   What are the similarities and differences between open and closed adoption?

7)   How did teen emancipation laws evolve in your community and state?

8)   How do teens commonly cope with the grief of abortion?

9)   Is it helpful to have a pregnant teen who has spontaneously miscarried continue to attend a support group for pregnant teens?

10)   Compare the costs of pregnancy and child-raising, open or closed adoption, and abortion.

MODULE SEVENTEEN
VIOLENCE AND TEEN SEXUALITY

"Victoria's Bad Rap"

Victoria came to us straight out of MTV. She was pierced with every imaginable body adornment. A black rose embellished the lateral aspect of her left ankle and from her navel hung a little pewter anchor. Outlining her ears were tiny rings capped with carnelian, topaz, emerald, and zircon. A large silver hoop hung like an exclamation point from her right earlobe.

Victoria's attraction was her candor and her long magenta fingernails as she talked about life, pregnancy, and death on the streets of San Francisco. Her virtual reality was the collapse of teen invincibility and none of us could counter her charge that, "My friends never live to see twenty, so what's the big deal about getting pregnant?"

I probably knew Victoria as well as any person who bounced between the fringes and the center of her life saga. We met one day when Mary Louise, her school counselor, was out of town and Victoria had an emergent need to see someone because her ulcer was activating itself. There is a refrain from a pop song that goes "some of them want to use you. . .some of them want to be used by you. . . some of them want to abuse you . . . some of them want to be abused." Victoria abused the good people in her life and sucked up to the abusers. It was a survival technique she had learned before kindergarten.

After eight months of running away, switching to alternative school, writing bad checks, and hanging out with the stoners and the druggies,   Victoria was back in high school telling me she wanted to start over. "Would you help?" she asked, and I said, "Of course, but you can't be playing games like before." She knew what I meant. "Okay", she said. Of course I didn't believe her; but I wasn't going to pull any support either, in case it might help.

We talked quite a bit during those next few weeks and she actually stayed in school through the spring. Victoria felt good because her San Francisco stepfather was going to be brought to justice. Victoria had never known her natural father and Victoria's mother settled with Mr. "Lookin Good" Willis because he had so many fine qualities - good looks, good clothes, good presentation. He gave Mama and her four kids a name, a house, a car, and a steady income. Then he went on to share his drinking problem with his new wife, rape her daughter, and molest her son. Nice!

In the midst of all the running away, someone began believing Victoria's incredible story. Victoria's first reaction was "Great, they will lock up the son-of-a-bitch and I will have Mama, Nick, and the twins back the way it used to be." Wrong! Mama and the gang sided in with "Everything's Goin' My Way" Willis. He did not go behind bars. He spent his month's vacation on house arrest with daily release time to attend sexual offender counseling at the local mental health center. He was back on the job and "cured" by the Fourth of July.

That fall, Victoria returned to school with a new identity; she was pregnant and she had a new last name. No, she was not married to Blaine, her boyfriend; she had taken her Mama's maiden name. Blaine was a senior at the high school across town and had finished vo-tech classes for a career as a flight mechanic. During the summer, Victoria and Blaine had dated at least a half a dozen times and were "in love" and "in hate" on a regular basis. Typically, Blaine acted like a stud and the next moment was denying fatherhood. For the last months of the pregnancy, Victoria stayed in school with adequate attendance and actually retained a fair grade point average.

Victoria rarely missed our weekly pregnancy support group meetings. Victoria's daughter Cassandra was a Christmas present, but half the time Victoria was ashamed of her. Cassandra had torticollis; the nerve that feeds the side of the face had been crushed during delivery leaving her face lopsided. It was not a permanent condition because the nerve readily regenerates in a healthy baby. "Sure, and hell is freezing over," Victoria would cynically counter when I told her the sides of Cassandra's face would become equal. Victoria kept on trying to be that "good mother" and to keep the same habits she had during the preceding nine months. But it was difficult; with the baby's schedule, school, and a part-time job plus Blaine's belligerence at fathering, Victoria's life was in a turmoil. Some days she would share her pain in the group. At other times, she would put on her happy face and I knew she was lying to herself.

Often Victoria's caretaking of her baby was outrageous; one day she did not want to wake up Cassandra while she stopped for a hamburger. She did not go by the drive-up window; but rather left the car running with the infant sleeping in the back seat of the car in mid-January weather. It was reported. The policeman found Victoria at AJ's, blithely chatting with her friends. Victoria was indignant about the circumstances when the officer handed her a ticket and asked Victoria to obtain an appointment with her social worker.

> **"To make the human connection in a loving relationship, say 'I Love You' often . . ."**

There was a poignant, touching side to Victoria born of well-camouflaged grief. We all prepared for a group presentation to kids at risk and afterward she read some of her poetry to us. I still have her handwritten notes from the presentation. They begin, "To make the human connection in a loving relationship, say 'I Love You' often . . ."

Victoria lost her place with Blaine; but Blaine's mom Julia took an interest in her granddaughter. Even when Victoria almost lost custody of Cassandra, Julia would come to visit them at the Last Chance Hotel where Victoria and Cassandra were living - temporarily. Victoria lived there until well after graduation.

The next fall, Victoria's life took a turn for the better. She was very happy and called saying she was the mother of two and she had a great boyfriend who had provided a house where she could start a day care. Mark was working so she could stay home with Cassy and also be a mother to his little boy. Mark and Victoria stopped by school one morning. She was radiant; her beautiful brown hair shown with its red highlights and abundant curls. Mark and Victoria were on their way to see their brother's new baby in San Francisco.

I never saw Victoria again and this morning I opened the paper and there it was - Mark admitting that he had killed Victoria and Cassy. I saw the picture of the shallow basement grave where they were buried. I thought about Victoria and Cassy and how they would get over hell and torticollis, and I cried.

CHALLENGE: The reader is challenged to write Module Seventeen and the goals and objectives for overcoming violence to teens and young children in the community.

SUGGESTIONS FOR CONSIDERATION:

1)   What do youngsters learn in a K-6 curriculum on conflict management that contributes to reducing the violence of abusive relationships, fighting, sexual harrassment, and bodily assault?

2)   Are characteristics of violence prevention present in the resilient youngster?

3)   We are well into the information age. With the explosion of knowledge and use of computers, what are the ramifications of violence education and prevention when considering video games, virtual reality, and cyber space?

4)   Is forgiving oneself a nonviolent action?

5)   Schools establish attendance policies that track tardies, absences, and dropouts. How is this helpful to violence prevention within a community?

6)   "Legal interventions impose academic, civil, and criminal penalties on certain unwanted behaviors to lower the risk of violence." If a teen has been drinking and becomes violent, are police force, restraints, and intimidation legal interventions? Do restraints and force deter violence? Under what circumstances do they aggravate a situation?

7)   Consider school sportsmanship, student uniforms, dress codes, faculty and student name tags, electronic monitors, closed circuit television, and metal detectors when writing goals about violence reduction and prevention.

8)   What does it mean to involve peers in violence mediation?

9)   It is characteristic of most teens to believe that they are invincible. Has the violence present in the hard drug culture made a difference in teens' perception of their invincibility?

10) Do current church and religious social leaders model nonviolence?

MODULE EIGHTEEN
GROUP CLOSURE

"Steps of Power"

Steps of Power

A lowly man, a puzzled man found something
    well before his time;
He fought it, he questioned it,
    he wondered day after day where he'd gone wrong.

Nothing wrong, after many trials convinced,
    he led an adventure against nothing wrong.
Now pleased with the idea he had stumbled upon,
    stepping toward power; he stepped toward the man he would find inside himself
        tomorrow.

Stepping toward love,
    he confided in it.
He longed for it when it felt far away;
    it cornered him, and he felt peace all about.

        He stepped to the top, mountains
        crossed, a humbled man.

Student Contribution

GOAL: To acknowledge the success of each group member and their family.

Objective One: Plan a picnic with invitations to all group members and their families.

Objective Two: Use a formal ceremony to acknowledge and share the pride of teen sexuality.

Objective Three: Give special recognition to pregnant teens who are graduating.

Objective Four: Allow time for grieving if a member is having difficulty with separation.

Objective Five: Reassure members with information about other community resources.

METHOD: Group closure is a time of sharing the goodness of who we are as sexual beings. A short formal ceremony that gives each member time to acknowledge and to be acknowledged is adequate. Some members may have prepared the gift of a card, a flower, a treat, a poem, or an inspirational message; whatever seems appropriate to the group members is acceptable.

Occasionally a group member has a difficult time grieving the loss of group support as he or she graduates or moves to a different community. Group members extend reassurance when they share and support continued contact.   Community agencies   are   helpful; nurse/social worker teams are   understanding, supportive, and do make home visits if a teen who is pregnant fears the ending of group   work.   Other members will be returning to the group as it opens in a community agency during the summer or when school starts in the new school year.

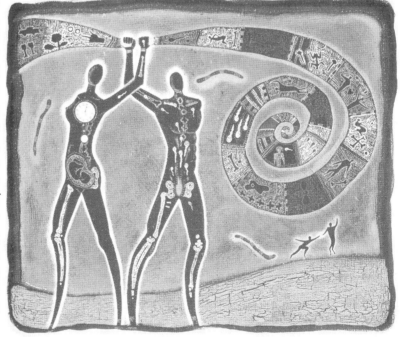

APPENDICES

GLOSSARY
OF REPRODUCTIVE ANATOMY AND RELATED TERMS

abruptio placenta - Premature and abrupt tearing of the placenta away from the wall of the womb where it is attached. A condition more apt to occur in teen pregnancy than in the pregnancy of a fully mature women.

abstinence - Choosing not to participate in the act of sexual intercourse.

acquired immunodeficiency syndrome (AIDS) - The incurable syndrome that is identified by a compromised immune system; a secondary infection is the actual cause of death because the immunity to fight disease is lost.

Aid to Families with Dependent Children (AFDC) - A federal entitlement program to needy families that meet federal poverty income guidelines.

amniotic sac, fluid - The fetal membranes which form a protective sac around the developing embryo; this sac, known as the "bag of water" fills with fluid to protect the embryo by cushioning shock and reducing heat loss.

anorexia - An eating disorder characterized by a distorted body image and the abhorrence of food which results in weight loss and the loss of monthly periods.

assertiveness - To appropriately express one's feelings so that personal rights and boundaries are not compromised.

ATOD - The acronym that means alcohol, tobacco, and other drugs.

bladder - The vessel that stores urine as it is processed by the kidney; the urethra in the male and female are the passageway from the bladder to the outside of the body for the excretion of urine.

Braxton-Hicks contractions - "False labor" or annoying short contractions that occur throughout pregnancy as the uterine muscle expands with the growth of the fetus.

bulimia - An eating disorder that is characterized by a distorted body image that demands the purging of food that has been ingested.

Carl-Perkins Vocational Grant - Funding source for vocational help to single pregnant and parenting high school students.

cervix - The mouth or opening of the womb or uterus.

Caesarean section - Surgical "birth of baby" through abdomen and womb; creates less stress with maternal or child complications.

codependency - Obsessing about or allowing another person's behavior to affect or control one's life.

confidentiality - The counselor-counselee relationship privilege that legally precludes disclosure.

consanguineous - Of the same blood.

CSAP - Acronym that stands for Center for Substance Abuse Prevention and is the governmental source of funds to help communities decrease alcohol and other drug abuse and the ensuing destruction of family systems when help and treatment is not available.

fallopian tube - The paired tubal organ on either side of the uterus that carries the egg from the ovary to the uterus.

fertilization - The union of the female ova and the male sperm in the body of the female.

fetus - The identity given to the unborn from the third month of gestation to delivery.

foreskin - The protective sheath of tissue surrounding all but the urethra of the penis; for reasons of ritual and cleanliness, the tissue is removed by a process called circumcision.

full-term - The full nine calendar months of a normal pregnancy; on a lunar calendar this is ten months or forty weeks. Preterm is an activity occurring before the end of the ninth month. Preterm labor would be commencement of labor before the end of the ninth month or before the fetus is fully formed and physically ready to live outside the womb.

gestation - Pregnancy; carrying the offspring from fertilization to birth.

grief loss - Any loss that can be identified by discreet stages of process. Teens often show cycles of loss during their pregnancy because they grieve life as it would have been were they not pregnant. They go through the cycle of grief - denial, bargaining, anger, and acceptance numerous times during pregnancy and parenting. These cycles can be because of loss of family expectation fulfillment, loss of body image, loss of teen identity, and loss of peer support.

group ground rules - Guidelines for group operation so all members are shown respect, support, and safety.

human chorionic gonadotropin (HCG) - The hormone secreted by the chorion or outer fetal membrane. Maternal blood levels of the hormone rise within a week to show a positive pregnancy test; morning urine levels of the hormone are detectable about a month after conception.

human immunodeficiency virus (HIV) - The virus, transmitted through the exchange of blood, semen, or vaginal discharge, that has the ability to attack and destroy the T-cells of the human body.

infant - A term that characterizes a child after birth to one year of age.

infant mortality - The number of infants per thousand population that die in their first year of life.

lactation - Production of milk.

licensed day care - Day care for working or student mothers that meets state requirements in areas of trained skilled child care, nutritious meals, safe and warm surroundings, and a stimulating educational environment.

low birth weight - A birth weight of less than five and one-half pounds. Birth weight is a key indicator of an infant's ability to survive and to thrive. Over one-half of babies who die are low birth weight. Of those babies that survive, low birth weight babies are ten times more likely to have learning problems in school.

menstruation - The monthly period or discharge of blood from the uterus through the vagina; the blood contains nutrients that accumulate on the wall of the womb or uterus in preparation for a fertilized egg; these nutrients are discharged if no pregnancy occurs.

nongonococcal urethritis (NGU) - An infection and inflammation of the male or female urethra that is identified by the discharge of purulent matter; however, the purulence is caused by an organism other than the gonococcus neisseria which causes gonorrhea.

outreach coordinator - The persons involved in reaching pregnant and parenting youth with information about the support and parenting programs.

ova - The female cell of reproduction.

ovary - The paired organ in a female where eggs and sex hormones are produced and stored.

ovulation - The discharge of an egg from the ovary; this process alternates from ovary to ovary each month.

penis - The male organ of intercourse.

perinatal - Events or conditions characterized by nativity or birth condition; events that surround a birth.

placenta - The bed that is connected by the umbilical cord to the baby for nutrient purpose; this "afterbirth" is expelled after birth of the baby.

postpartum - After delivery.

prenatal - Existing or happening before birth. For instance, the information that a prospective mother receives from health care professionals is called prenatal education.

prostate - The organ surrounding the neck of the bladder and the urethra in the male; its functions are not fully understood.

psychoses - Mental disorders characterized by the inability to receive, interpret, and communicate reality in a "normal" manner.

rectum - The last section of the alimentary canal or gastrointestinal tract. Stool is stored in the rectum before it passes to the outside of the body through the anus.

reproduction - To produce; to bear offspring.

scrotum- The sac that carries the testes.

secondary virginity - The idea of forgiving oneself if there is guilt over the loss of virginity.

self-efficacy - Knowing and feeling control of oneself and one's environment. Colloquially known as a "can-do" spirit.

self-worth - A term used to denote valuing one's self as a person; can be used interchangeably with self-esteem.

seminal vesicle - The vessel connected to the duct through which semen reaches the penis for ejaculation.

Serenity Prayer - The prayer of St. Francis of Assisi that is widely used in self-help groups as their personal growth allows them "the Serenity to accept the things I cannot change, the Courage to change the things I can, and the Wisdom to know the difference."

sexually transmitted diseases (STD) - Any disease contracted through sexual intercourse or its accompanying behaviors.

sperm- The male cell of reproduction.

Teen Parents: Reachable/Teachable - A name for the concept of support and empowerment of the pregnant and parenting teen.

teratogens - Chemical substances injurious or lethal to a developing fetus.

testicle - The male reproductive gland that carries the sperm cells.

umbilical cord - The tissue that surrounds and strengthens the vessels that carry blood to and from the mother and the fetus.

uterus - The womb or enclosure that envelopes the fertilized egg; the egg develops into a fetus and the fetus develops into a full term baby.

urethra - The canal through which urine is passed from the bladder to the outside of the body.

vagina - The canal that leads from the uterus to the outside of a woman's body; it is located between the urethra and the anus; it is also the channel through which the baby is delivered.

vas deferens - The excretory duct of the testes.

Women, Infants, and Children (WIC) - A federally funded food supplement program that helps reduce low birth weight babies and increase full term gestation through good nutrition to women, infants, and children.

REFERENCES

Overview
Corey, G., Corey, M.S. (1987). *Groups: Process and Practice*. Pacific Grove, California: Brooks/Cole Publishing Company.

Corey, G., Corey, M.S., Callanan, P.J., Russell, J.M. (1988). *Group Techniques*. Pacific Grove, California: Brooks/Cole Publishing Company.

Module One - Introduction
Jung, C.G. (1973). *Four Archtypes*. Princeton, New Jersey: Princeton University Press.

Kids Count Data Book (1995). Washington D.C., The Annie B. Casey Foundation and Center for the Study of Social Policy.

Morris, L., Warren, C.W., Aral, S.O. (1993). Measuring Adolescent Sexual Behaviors and Related Health Outcomes, *Public Health Reports*, *108*, 31-35.

Rathus, S.A., Nevid, J. S. (1991) *Abnormal Psychology*. Englewood Cliffs, New Jersey: Prentice-Hall, Inc., 42-43.

Module Two - Puberty
Mayle, P. (1989). *What's Happening To Me?* New York, New York: Carol Publishing Group.

Mayo, M.A. (1991). *Mom's A Bird, Dad's A Bee*. Eugene, Oregon: Harvest House Publishers.

Module Three - The Health Questionnaire and The Genogram As Interview Tools
Agee, J. (1941). *Now Let Us Praise Famous Men*. Boston, Massachusetts: Houghton-Mifflin Company.

Bradshaw, J. (1988). *Bradshaw On: The Family*. Pompano Beach, Florida: Health Communications, Inc.

Djerassi C. (1992). *The Pill, Pygmy Chimps, and Degas' Horse*. New York, New York: BasicBooks.

Doctorow, E. L. (1976). *Ragtime*. New York, New York: Random House.

George, R.L. (1990). *Counseling The Chemically Dependent*. Needham Heights, Massachusetts: Allyn and Bacon.

Kitzinger, S., Bailey, V. (1993). *Pregnancy Day By Day*. New York, New York: Alfred A. Knopf.

Maslow, A. (1970). *Motivation and Personality*, New York, New York: Harper and Row.

Praeger, S.G., Martin, L.S. (1994). Using Genogram and Ecomaps In Schools, *Journal of School Nursing, 10,* 34-40.

University of Colorado Health Sciences Center (1988). *Genetic Applications.* Lawrence, Kansas: Learner Managed Designs Publications.

Wegscheider, S. (1981). *Another Chance.* Palo Alto, California: Science and Behavior Books.

Wegscheider-Cruse, S., Cruse, J.R. (1990). *Understanding Codependency.* Deerfield Beach, California: Health Communications, Inc.

Module Four - Group Ground Rules
Corey, G., Corey, M.S. (1987). *Groups: Process and Practice.* Pacific Grove, California: Brooks/Cole Publishing Company.

Corey, G., Corey, M.S., Callanan, P. (1988). *Issues and Ethics In The Helping Professions.* Pacific Grove, California: Brooks/Cole Publishing Company, 189-191, 201.

Melroe, H.N. (1990). Duty to Warn Versus Patient Confidentiality, *Nurse Practitioner, 2,* 58-69.

Module Five - Cookie Bake And Career Night
Lewis, C.S. (1960). *The Four Loves.* New York, New York: Harcourt, Brace, and World, Inc.

Molineux, B. (1996). The Four Types of Love, *The Good Enough Family.* Helena, Montana: Independent Record.

Module Six - Using The Mandala
Acts, Psalms, *The Holy Bible: Revised Standard Version* (1962). New York, New York: The World Publishing Company.

Argulles, J., Argulles, M. (1972). *Mandala.* excerpt from *Black Elk Speaks.* Boulder, Colorado: Shambhala Publications, Inc.

I Ching, Book of Changes (1967). Translated by Wilhelm, R., Baynes, C.F. for Bollingen Foundation, Princeton, New Jersey: Princeton University Press.

Jung, C.J. (1964) *Man and His Symbols.* New York, New York: Doubleday.

Morris, S.W. (1993). Designing Health Promotion Approaches to High Risk Adolescents Through Formative Research with Youth and Parents, *Public Health Reports*, 108, 68-77.

Niehardt, J.G. (1993). *Black Elk Speaks.* Lincoln, Nebraska: University of Nebraska Press.

Module Seven - Assertiveness

Allport, G.W. (1937) *Personality of Psychological Interpretation*. New York, New York: Holt.

Cantor, D.W., Bernay, T., Stoess, J. (1992). *Women In Power,* New York, New York: Houghton-Mifflin Company.

Erikson, E.H. (1963). *Childhood and Society*. New York, New York: W.W. Norton and Co., Inc.

Erikson, E.H. (1963). Stages of Development, (from Rathus and Nevid. 1991). Englewood Cliffs, New Jersey: Prentice-Hall, Inc.

Foon, A.E. (1986). Effect of Locus of Control on Counseling Expectations of Clients, *Journal of Counseling Psychology, 33*, 4, 462-464.

Lerner, H.G. (1985). *The Dance of Anger*. New York, New York: Harper and Row, Inc.

McCormick, I.A., Walkey, F.H. (1984). Reliability and Normative Data for the Simple Rathus Assertiveness Schedule, *New Zealand Journal of Psychology, 13,*69-70.

McCullagh, J.G. (1982). Assertiveness Training for Boys in Junior High School, *Social Work Education, 5,1,* 41-51.

Pipher, M. (1994). *Reviving Ophelia*. New York, New York: Ballintine Books.

Rathus, S.A. (1973). A 30-Item Schedule for Assessing Assertive Behavior, *Behavior Therapy, 4,* 398-406.

Rathus, S.A., Nevid, J.S. (1977). Concurrent Validity of the 30-Item Assertiveness Schedule With a Psychiatric Population, *Behavior Therapy, 8,* 393-397.

Robinson, W.L., Calhoun, K.S. (1984). Assertiveness and Cognitive Processing in Interpersonal Relationships, *Journal of Behavioral Therapy, 6,* 1.

Rotter, J.B. (1966). Generalized Expectancies for Internal versus External Control of Reinforcement, *Psychological Monographs, 80,1,*609.

Rotter, J.B. (1954). *Social Learning and Clinical Theory,* Englewood Cliffs, New Jersey: Prentice-Hall, Inc.

Werner-Davis, M. (1992). *Divorce Busting*. New York, New York: A Fireside Book.

Wolpe, J, Lazarus, A.A. (1966). *Behavior Therapy Techniques,* New York, New York: Pergamon Press.

Module Eight - Alcohol, Tobacco, Drug Use And Abuse

Arthurs, K. (1996). ADD Update: Dealing with attention deficit disorder naturally. *Health Counselor, 8,* 16-18.

Finke, L., Chorpenning, J., French, B., Leese, C., Siegel, M. (1996). Drug and Alcohol Use of School-Age Children in a Rural Community. *Journal of School Nursing, 12,* 10-13.

George, R.L. (1990). *Counseling The Chemically Dependent.* Needham Heights, Massachusetts: Allyn and Bacon.

McAuliffe, R.M., McAuliffe, M.B. (1985). *Essentials For The Diagnosis Of Chemical Dependency,* Minneapolis, Minnesota: The American Chemical Dependency Society.

Module Nine - Self-Worth And Codependency

American Psychiatric Association (1994). *Diagnostic and Statistical Manual of Mental Disorders,* (Fourth Edition) Washington, D.C.

Beattie, M. (1987). *Codependent No More,* New York, New York: HarperCollins Publishers.

Walters, L.H., Walters, J., McHenry, P. (1986). Differentiation of Girls at Risk of Early Pregnancy from the General Population of Adolescents, *Journal of Genetic Psychology, 148,* 19-29.

Module Ten - Birth Control And Sexually Transmitted Diseases

Alan Guttmacher Institute (1991). *Fact In Brief: Teenage Sexual and Reproductive Behavior,* New York, New York.

Allen, T. (1994). Will Kids Buy Abstinence?, *Education Digest,* from *Virginia Journal of Education, 88,* 6-12

Brochures and Handouts adapted for National Association of High School Student Council Representatives, "Birth Control, Which Contraceptive Method Is Best For You?," "Birth Control Methods and Effectiveness," "Sex and the Single Teen," and "A Quick Index of Sexually Transmitted Diseases," (1990). New York, New York: Planned Parenthood.

Gingess, P. (1989). Evaluation of Training Effects on Teacher Attitudes and Concerns Prior to Implementing a Human Sexuality Education Program, *Journal of School Health, 4,* 156-160.

Gordon, D.E. (1990). Formal Operational Thinking: The Role of Cognitive-Developmental Processes in Adolescent Decision-Making About Pregnancy and Contraception, *American Journal of Orthopsychiatry, 60,* 3.

Lawrence, L., Levy, S.R., Robinson, L. (1990). Self-efficacy and AIDS Prevention for Pregnant Teens, *Journal of School Health, 60,* 19-24.

Ross, M.W., Caudle, C., Taylor, J. (1989). A Preliminary Study of Social Issues in AIDS Prevention Among Adolescents, *Journal of School Health, 59,* 308-311.

Williams, J.M., Stout, J.K. (1984). The Effect of High and Low Assertiveness on Locus of Control and Health Problems, *The Journal of Psychology, 119, 2,* 169-173.

Module Eleven - Hormones, Humor, And Good Grief
Cousins, N. (1985). *Anatomy Of An Illness,* New York, New York: A Bantam Book.

Berliner, D. (1995). *Handbook of Educational Psychology.* New York, New York: MacMillan Publishing Company.

Gonick, L. (1995). Science Classics: Pheroflying. *Discover,* 75-76.

Kubler-Ross, E. (1969). *On Death And Dying.* New York, New York: MacMillan Publishing Company, Inc.

Rando, T. (1984). *Grief, Death, And Dying,* Champaign, Illinois: Research Press Company.

Module Twelve - Gestation, Labor And Delivery, Preterm Labor
Ali, S. E. (1995) *Cultures Of The World, Afghanistan.* White Plains, New York: Marshall Cavendish Corporation.

Bradley, R. A. (1994). *Gestation, A Video About the First Days of Life.* Sherman Oaks, California: Academy Communications.

Colberg, J.O. (1971). *Where Are You Mohammed Khan?* Unpublished: Author.

Curtis, G.B. (1994). *Your Pregnancy Week By Week.* Tuscon, Arizona: Fisher Books.

Hotchner, T. (1992). *The Pregnancy Diary,* New York, New York: Avon Books.

Kitzinger, S., Bailey, V. (1993). *Pregnancy Day By Day.* New York, New York: Alfred A. Knopf.

Mayle, P., Robins, A. (1977). *Where Did I Come From?* New York, New York: Carol Publishing Group.

Nilsson, L., Hamberger, L. (1993). *A Child Is Born.* New York, New York: Delacorte Press.

Nilsson, L., Swanberg, L. (1994). *How Was I Born?* New York, New York: Delacorte Press.

Robinson, K. (1993). The Support Needs of Pregnant and Parenting High School Students, *Journal of School Nursing, 9,* 12-15.

Simkin, P., Whaley, J., Keppler, A. (1991). *Pregnancy, Childbirth, and The New Born,* New York, New York: Meadowbrook Press.

Module Thirteen - Nutrition

Healthy People 2000. (1991). *National Health Promotion and Disease Prevention Objectives.* Washington, DC: U.S. Department of Health and Human Services.

Sears, B. (1995). *The Zone: A Dietary Roadmap,* New York, New York: Regan Books.

Smith, L. (1981). *Foods For Healthy Kids,* New York, New York: McGraw-Hill Book Company.

Weiss, L., Katzman, M., Wolchik, S. (1985). *Treating Bulimia: A Psychoeducational Approach,* Elmford, New York: Pergamon Press, Inc.

Module Fourteen - Male Responsibility, Father Bonding

Wright, R. (1994). *The Moral Animal.* New York, New York: Pantheon Books.

Elsters, A.B., Lamb, M.E., Kimmberly, N. (1983). Perceptions of Parenthood Among Adolescent Fathers, *Pediatrics,* 758-765.

Horn, W.F. (1995). *Father Facts,* Lancaster, Pennsylvania: National Fatherhood Initiative.

Module Fifteen - Preparing For Child Care

Colberg, J.O. (1991). *A Study of School Policy and Drop-Out Rates Among Pregnant Teens in a Rural Setting,* Unpublished: Author.

Crouch, J.G. (1989). Perceived Child-Rearing Dimensions and Assertiveness, *Adolescence, 24,* 93.

Edwards, L.E. (1977). An Experimental Comprehensive High School Clinic, *American Journal of Public Health, 67,* 8.

Furstenberg, F.F. (1987). Adolescent Mothers and Their Children in Later Life, *Family Relations, 40,* 142-151.

Ortman, P.E., (1988). Adolescents' Perceptions of and about Control and Responsibility in Their Lives, *Adolescence, 23,* 92.

Vincent, M.L., Clearie, A.F., Schluchter, M.D. (1987). Reducing Adolescent Pregnancy Through School and Community-Based Education. *Journal of the American Medical Association, 257,* 3382-3386.

Module Sixteen - Other Pregnancy Outcomes

DuPrau, J. (1990). *Adoption,* Englewood Cliffs, New Jersey: Messner Publishing Co.

Lindsay, J.W., *Open Adoption: A Caring Option,* Buena Park, California: Morning Glory Press.

Silber, K., Speedlin, P. (1991). *Dear Birthmother.* San Antonio, Texas: Corona Publishing Company.

Module Seventeen - Violence And Teen Sexuality
Barbour, S., Swisher, K., eds. (1996). *Violence: Opposing Viewpoint,* San Diego, California: Greenhaven Press, Inc.

Beck, A.T., Ward, C.H., Mendelson, M., Mock, J., Erbaugh, J. (1961). An Inventory For Measuring Depression, *Archives of General Psychiatry, 4,* 561-571.

Boyer, D., Fine, D. (1992). Sexual Abuse as a Factor in Adolescent Pregnancy. *Family Planning Perspectives, 24,* 4.

Woodson, J. (1995). *Autobiography of a Family Photo,* New York, New York: Penguin Books.
Module Eighteen - Group Closure
Corey, G., Corey, M.S. (1987). *Groups: Process and Practice.* Pacific Grove, California: Brooks/Cole Publishing Company.

Corey, G., Corey, M.S., Callahan, P.J., Russell, J.M. (1988). *Group Techniques.* Pacific Grove, California: Brooks/Cole Publishing Company.

CURRENT STATISTICS

We explore teen sexualization in order to reduce teen pregnancy. Because there are many hidden facts and feelings, statistics are helpful to point us in the right direction. We need to trust our judgment about a problem in light of what we see. In other words, just because statistics present an epidemic picture, do not view the issue as immense beyond the management skills or resources in your family, school, church, or community.

Every state contributes their information on adolescent pregnancy and other behavioral indicators to the Center for the Study of Social Policy and the Annie E. Casey Foundation which publish the *Kids Count Data Book*. The *Kids Count Data Book* uses the ten following indicators to synthesize a statistical picture of American youth and their dilemma: 1) percentage of low birth weight babies, 2) infant mortality rate, 3) child death rate, 4) percentage of all birth that are to pregnant teens, 5) juvenile violent crime arrest rate, 6) percentage graduating from high school, 7) percentage of teens not in school and not in labor force, 8) teen violent death rate, 9) percentage of children in poverty, and 10) percentage of children in single parent homes.

Each day in America about 20,000 women get pregnant. Approximately 3000 or about 13% of this number are teenagers. About one-half of the teens give birth; the other half miscarry or have abortions. Each day about 8000 teens become sexually active and each day 1500 drop out of school. Can you make a difference in these statistics?

"PROGRAM HISTORY AND STATISTICS FOR RED LIGHT, GREEN LIGHT"

The teen pregnancy prevention program described in *Red Light, Green Light* grew out of a peer support group approach to help pregnant and parenting students attain academic, vocational, and social success without leaving the normal high school setting. The program also promoted prevention of a second pregnancy in the teen years. Of the one-hundred and sixty-nine pregnant students served from 1988 to 1995 there were thirteen repeat pregnancies in the teen years. The prevention component of the program was studied and out of that study grew the basis for the book, *Red Light, Green Light*.

In 1987, administrators and the school nurse determined that about fifteen students had dropped out of high school because support services were not available for pregnant and parenting teens. In 1988, ninety-eight students were given a questionnaire that explored attendance, academic standing, health status, and willingness to take part in a support group, affirming a desire to stay in school and graduate. All participants had good attendance records, and grade point averages ranged between 3.5 to 1.9. Forty-five students, with their parents' permission, opted to take part in a pilot program; of the forty-five, twenty-six were pregnant and of those twenty-six, only three dropped out of school. Using information learned from this control group, the school implemented the program in the 1988-89 school year.

The support group format encourages teens to identify their own needs and operate "by teens for teens." Students are not "coerced to take on someone else's emotionality but rather are prompted to investigate their own family values and patterns of emotional expression." The program supports good communication with parents and disseminates information about prevention to civic groups, local health departments, private medical clinics, family planning agencies, the faith community, and social service agencies.

Presently, state and district funding enables a self-contained program of parenting and child care to exist outside of high school in an alternative area. The program described in *Red Light, Green Light* continues as a prevention model and as an outreach program to teens in high school.

RESOURCE GUIDE

Alan Guttmacher Institute
2010 Massachusetts Avenue NW
Washington, DC 20063
 Established institute for information and statistics on teen pregnancy and prevention.

American Academy of Pediatrics
Division of Publications
141 Northwest Point Boulevard
P.O. Box 927
Elk Grove, Illinois 60009-0927
 Brochures on child and adolescent health concerns.

Annie E. Casey Foundation
One Lafayette Place
Greenwich, Connecticutt 06830
(203) 661-2773, FAX (203) 661-5127
 Copublisher of *Kids Count Data Book.*

Baby Think It Over
P.O. Box 64184
Tacoma, Washington 98466
Voice/Fax (206)582-BABY
 Information about a realistic infant simulator designed by current parents for future parents.

Center for Population Options
1012 Fourteenth Street NW
Washington, DC 20005
 Statistical information on adolescent sexuality. Monitors changes in state laws.

Center for the Study of Social Policy
1250 Eye Street NW, Suite 503
Washington, DC 20005
(202) 371-1565, FAX (202) 371-1472
 Copublisher of *Kids Count Data Book.*

Community of Caring
1350 New York Avenue, NW, Suite 500
Washington, DC 20005-4709
(202) 393-1250
 Information and training about community networks to support the welfare of children.

Consumer Information Catalog
Consumer Information Center T
P.O. Box 100
Pueblo, Colorado 81002
    Free catalog of information available from CIC

CSAP National Resource Center
Center for Substance Abuse Prevention
9302 Lee Highway
Fairfax, Virginia 22031
(703) 218-5700, FAX (703) 218-5701, 1-800-354-8824
    Free information on materials and programs to prevent perinatal drug and alcohol abuse.

Education For Parenting
31 West Coulter Street
Philadelphia, Pennsylvania 19144
(215) 438-1255, (215) 438-1380
    A very young person's program to learn responsibility and caring.

Far West Laboratory for Educational Research and Development
730 Harrison Street
San Francisco, California 94107-1242
    Investigates new educational programs, ideas, and philosophies.

Florence Crittenton Division
Child Welfare League of America
67 Irving Place
New York, New York 10003
    Program information for teen mothers.

Focus On The Family
P.O. Box 500
Arcadia, California 91006-0500
  Helpful information pamphlets specific to pregnant teens.

Growing Up Caring
P.O. Box 9509
15319 Chatsworth Street
Mission Hills, California 91395-9509
  Students caring for themselves and caring for others.

Growing Up Christian In a Sexy World
Pastor Ken Moore, Coordinator
First Christian Church
311 Power Street
Helena, Montana 59601
    Preteen program adapted from a book by the same name.

GRADS Program
American Home Economics Association
2010 Massachusetts Avenue NW
Washington, DC 20036-1028
    Complete program of ideas and activities for the high school pregnant and parenting teen.

Johnson and Johnson Consumer Products
P.O. Box 1112
Somerville, New Jersey 08876
  Free baby products, booklets, and handouts.

March Of Dimes
1275 Mamaroneck Avenue
White Plains, New York 10605
(914) 997-4792
    Catalog of free books, pamphlets, flyers, and videos on prevention, pregnancy, and parenting.

Morning Glory Press
6595 S.San Haroldo Way
Bueno Park, California 90620-3748
(714) 828-1998
    Publishing company specializing in books on concerns of teen sexuality and teen pregnancy.

National Organization on Adolescent Pregnancy and Parenting
P.O. Box 2365
Reston, Virginia 22090
  Write for membership information.

National Aids Information Clearinghouse
P.O. Box 6003
Rockville, Maryland 20850
1-900-458-5231

National Drug Abuse Hotline
1-800-COCAINE

National Fatherhood Initiative (NFI)
600 Eden Road, Building E
Lancaster, Pennsylvania 17601
(717) 581-8860 or FAX (717) 581-8862
> National non-profit organization dedicated to promoting responsible fatherhood in America.

Network Publications ETR Associates
1700 Mission Street, Suite 203
P.O. Box 8506
Santa Cruz, California 95061-8506
> Pamphlets on teen health and sexuality-related concerns.

Ortho Pharmaceutical Corporation
Department of Educational Services
Rartan, New Jersey 08869
> Free information on contraceptives and birth control methods.

Planned Parenthood
810 Seventh Avenue
New York, New York 10019
> Free catalog about items available through Planned Parenthood.

Proctor and Gamble
On Target Media, Inc.
Cincinatti, Ohio
> Offers comprehensive study handouts called *Childbirth Classroom.*

Southwest Regional Laboratory
4665 Lampson Avenue
Los Alamitos, California 90720
> Investigates new educational programs, ideas, and philosophies.

Sunburst
101 Castleton Street
Pleasantville, New York 10570-1207
1-800-431-1934
> Free catalog of videos available on teen concerns such as rape, alcohol, tobacco, drug abuse.

Teen Parents: Reachable/Teachable
Summer Kitchen Press
314 Chaucer Street
Helena, Montana 59601
1-800-418-5237
> Information about a support program for empowering pregnant and parenting teens.

The Center for Child and Family Studies
College of Social Work, University of South Carolina
Columbia, South Carolina 29208
(803) 777-9400
> Community networking ideas for the management of teen support groups.

The Center for Early Adolescence
University of North Carolina
Carr Mill Hall
Carrboro, North Carolina 27510
> Information that serves the preteen and the teen.

U.S. Department of Health and Human Services
Administration for Children, Youth, Family
Washington, DC 20201
> Teen parenting information.

Western Regional Center, Drug-Free Schools and Communities
Northwest Regional Educational Laboratory
101 SW Main Street, Suite 500
Portland, Oregon 97204
> Investigates new educational programs, ideas, and philosophies.

Young Families Support Program
Boston City Hospital, Adolescent Center ACC-2
818 Harrison Avenue
Boston, Massachusetts 02118
> Information about a program that serves adolescent mothers affected by substance abuse.

PREGNANCY CHECK LIST

Pregnancy Checklist	Date
1. Name	
2. Birth date	
3. Interview date	
4. Due date	
5. Last period	
6. Positive pregnancy test	
7. Parents notified	
8. Boyfriend notified	
9. Health pregnancy services notified	
10. 1st trimester follow-up	
11. Family planning	
12. Women Infants and Children (WIC)	
13. Medicaid (AFDC)	
14. Support group	
15. Counselor notified	
16. Teachers notified	
17. Nutrition	
18. Exercise	
19. Father responsibility	
20. 2nd trimester follow-up	
21. Private counselor	
22. Substance abuse	
23. Class flex-time	
24. Academic progress	
25. Abuse/violence	
26. Child care	
27. Prepared child birth	
28. School leave	
29. Breast feeding	
30. 3rd trimester follow-up	

"ABOUT THE AUTHOR"

Janet Ollila Colberg, RN, MHS, LPC, has worked as a high school nurse for eighteen years in Helena, Montana. Her master's degree is in counseling with licensure as a professional counselor in private practice. She is involved with the statewide workshops "Families and Youth In Crisis" and "Caring for Kids." Janet has also presented workshops for the Western Regional Center for Drug-Free Schools and Communities and the National Association of School Nurses.

"ABOUT THE ILLUSTRATOR"

Joel Nakamura, painter and illustrator, uses iconography and narrative symbolism to make his work fascinating. The figure is central, showing a unique depiction of man and his roles. Stripped away is the facade. The veneers of gender or race are removed, revealing an interior structure or dialogue. Thoughts, bones, and objects take on psychological and conceptual undertones. The images ask questions and sometimes answer them.

"WHAT'S IN A TITLE?"

The title of this book, *Red Light, Green Light*, is symbolic of the nature of teen sexuality and teen pregnancy. First, it symbolizes the stop and go nature of unspoken signals between teen women and their partners.

Second, it symbolizes the confusing messages that parents give their children when there are discrepancies between adult life styles and spoken messages.

Third, it is symbolic of the funding to support or to retract support of programs that are alternately high priority or not prioritized at all with reference to teen sexuality and teen pregnancy as an American societal concern.

Last, *Red Light, Green Light* symbolizes the commitment of communities or the withdrawal of support because the nature of teen behaviors is often hidden and difficult to remedy. Meeting adolescent needs requires cooperation of families and community services. Individuals and representatives of agencies put aside differences in the spirit of coming together for the good of all adolescents in the community.

ORDER FORM

RED LIGHT, GREEN LIGHT: Preventing Teen Pregnancy

Quantity _____ x Price/book* _____ = Amount _____

Shipping and Handling ($1.00/book, $3.00 minimum) _____

Total (Please enclose Check or Purchase Order with your order.) _____

*Price/book Quantity Discounts:
$14.50 each
Call for wholesale discounts.

Make checks payable to: SUMMER KITCHEN PRESS
Send orders to: Summer Kitchen Press
314 Chaucer Street
Helena, MT 59601
Phone: 1-800-418-5237

Ship to:
Name: _____

Organization: _____

Address: _____

_____

City: _____

State: _____ Zip Code: _____

Phone No.: _____ FAX: _____